Oestrogen Deficiency

Causes and Consequences

Advances
in Reproductive
Endocrinology

VOLUME 8

Oestrogen Deficiency

Causes and Consequences

Edited by RW Shaw

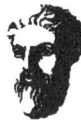

The Parthenon Publishing Group
International Publishers in Medicine, Science & Technology

Casterton Hall, Carnforth,
Lancs, LA6 2LA, UK

One Blue Hill Plaza, Pearl River,
New York 10965, USA

Published in the USA by
The Parthenon Publishing Group Inc.
One Blue Hill Plaza
PO Box 1564, Pearl River
New York 10965, USA

Published in the UK by
The Parthenon Publishing Group Limited
Casterton Hall, Carnforth
Lancs. LA6 2LA, England

Library of Congress Cataloging-in-Publication Data
Oestrogen deficiency: causes and consequences / edited by R.W. Shaw.
    p.   cm. — (Advances in reproductive endocrinology ; v. 8)
    "Proceedings of a meeting held at Warren House, Kingston-on-
Thames, UK, 26-27 June 1996."
    Includes bibliographical references and index.
    ISBN 1-852070-719-7
    1. Menopause—Complications—Congresses. 2. Estrogen—Physiological
effect—Congresses. 3. Menopause—Hormone therapy—Congresses.
I. Shaw Robert W. (Robert Wayne) II. Series.
    [DNLM: 1. Estrogens—deficiency—congresses. W1 AD83S v.8 1996 /
WP 522 029 1996]
RG186.028 1996
618.1'75—dc20
DNLM/DLC
for Library of Congress   96-16860
                                                                        CIP

British Library Cataloguing in Publication Data
Oestrogen deficiency : causes and consequences. – (Advances in reproductive
    endocrinology series ; v. 8)
    1. Menopause 2. Estrogen – Therapeutic use
    I. Shaw, Robert W. (Robert Wayne)
618.1'75

ISBN 1-85070-719-7

Typeset by Martin Lister Publishing Services, Carnforth, Lancs., UK
Printed and bound in the UK by Bookcraft (Bath) Ltd., Midsomer Norton, UK

Contents

List of principal contributors

D.H. Barlow
Nuffield Department of
 Obstetrics and Gynaecology
John Radcliffe Hospital
Maternity Department
Headington
Oxford OX3 9DU

J.E. Compston
Department of Medicine
University of Cambridge Clinical
 School
Level 5
Addenbrooke's Hospital
Hills Road
Cambridge CB2 2QQ

I. Fogelman
Department of Nuclear Medicine
Guy's Hospital
St. Thomas Street
London SE1 9RT

G.D.O. Lowe
Haemostasis, Thrombosis and
 Vascular Medicine Unit
Department of Medicine
Royal Infirmary
10 Alexandra Parade
Glasgow G31 2ER

D.W. Purdie
Centre for Metabolic Bone
 Disease
Alderson House
Hull Royal Infirmary
Anlaby Road
Hull HU3 2JZ

D. Ross
Wynn Institute for Metabolic
 Research
Cecil Rosen Research
 Laboratories
21 Wellington Road
London NW8 9SQ

R.W. Shaw
Department of Obstetrics and
 Gynaecology
University of Wales College of
 Medicine
Heath Park
Cardiff CF4 4XN

J.C. Stevenson
Wynn Institute for Metabolic
 Research
Cecil Rosen Research
 Laboratories
21 Wellington Road
London NW8 9SQ

D.W. Sturdee
Department of Obstetrics and
 Gynaecology
Solihull Hospital
Lode Lane
Solihull
West Midlands B91 2JL

M.P. Vessey
Department of Public Health and
 Primary Care
Gibson Building
Radcliffe Infirmary
Oxford OX2 6HE

Foreword

It is now apparent that the consequences of oestrogen deficiency extend far beyond the characteristic symptoms experienced at the menopause. These symptoms, whilst acute and severe for many individuals, tend to regress with time, albeit in some patients' last years.

The effects of withdrawal of the normal premenopausal circulating levels of oestradiol-17β, have now been shown to result in changes in many other systems. These include changes in serum lipids and their subfractions; haematological and clotting parameters; the cardiovascular system – particularly effects on the endothelial lining and smooth muscle responsiveness to contractility; and of course the long-term detrimental effects on bone mineral density with attendant increased fracture risk.

This monograph explores these issues in depth and extends discussion far beyond the topic of hormone replacement therapy to encompass the wider sphere of oestrogen deficiency occurring in association with amenorrhoea, premature ovarian failure following surgical oophorectomy and that associated with various drug therapies. The role of long-term replacement therapy, its potential disadvantages and health economic implications were also reviewed.

The proceedings are a distillate of presentations and discussions at a workshop of clinicians – gynaecologists, endocrinologists and physicians – and scientists sponsored by an educational grant from Zeneca Pharma UK and held in June 1995. It should provide an informative update and review for all those involved in the assessment and management of the increasing proportion of women with absent ovarian function and be of value in planning their assessment and management.

April 1996

Professor Robert W. Shaw
Head Dept. Obstetrics & Gynaecology
University of Wales
College of Medicine
Cardiff CF4 4XN
UK

1

Clinical symptoms of oestrogen deficiency

D. W. Sturdee

INTRODUCTION

It is not without good reason that the phrase 'the change of life' has been applied by women to the time of transition from normal pre-menopausal ovarian function to that of ovarian failure in the post-menopause. During this climacteric, the last period (menopause) will have different implications for women depending on their culture and tradition. In societies where menstruation is seen as polluting, Muslim women are in purdah, the release from such inferior status allows them to assume a new, important and rewarding role within the family and society. In contrast, modern Western societal values and attitudes are more likely to emphasize the negative aspects such as loss of femininity and sexual attractiveness. This time may also coincide with domestic changes such as children leaving home, parents becoming aged and infirm and husband at a stressful peak of his career, all of which may influence the way a woman adjusts to the climacteric and menopause. Ageing in itself is accompanied by various inevitable physical changes, and together with all these other aspects it can be difficult to determine which clinical symptoms are a result of oestrogen deficiency.

Epidemiological studies have shown that over 80% of women in the United Kingdom will experience some symptoms considered to be due to oestrogen deficiency during the climacteric[1]. Hot flushes

Table 1 Frequency of symptoms in 135 women attending a menopause clinic who had experienced a spontaneous menopause

Symptom	%
Hot flushes	75
Sweats	71
Lethargy	68
Loss of libido	65
Tension/irritability	65
Insomnia	64
Anxiety	62
Headaches	62
Muscular/joint pains	61
Depression	60
Hair/skin changes	58
Loss memory/concentration	53
Dry vagina	48
Fears ageing/health	47
Loss confidence	47
Weight gain	45
Indigestion/nausea	45
Dyspareunia	44
Palpitations/dizziness	44
Backache	39
Formication	33
Loss femininity	32
Urinary symptoms	30

and sweats are the most characteristic and common symptoms of the climacteric in the Western world, and of those experiencing a spontaneous menopause 60–75% will be affected[1-3]. In Japan, however, flushes are rarely experienced by menopausal women and there is not even a word in the Japanese language for it[4].

It is generally accepted that an induced menopause by surgical castration, chemotherapy or irradiation results in an even higher incidence of flushing, and with increased severity[5,6]. In most women these symptoms may persist for more than 1 year and in about a quarter for more that 5 years[1]. Parenthetically, men do not experience a comparable climacteric but following the uncommon event of testicular failure or bilateral orchidectomy, severe hot flushes and

2

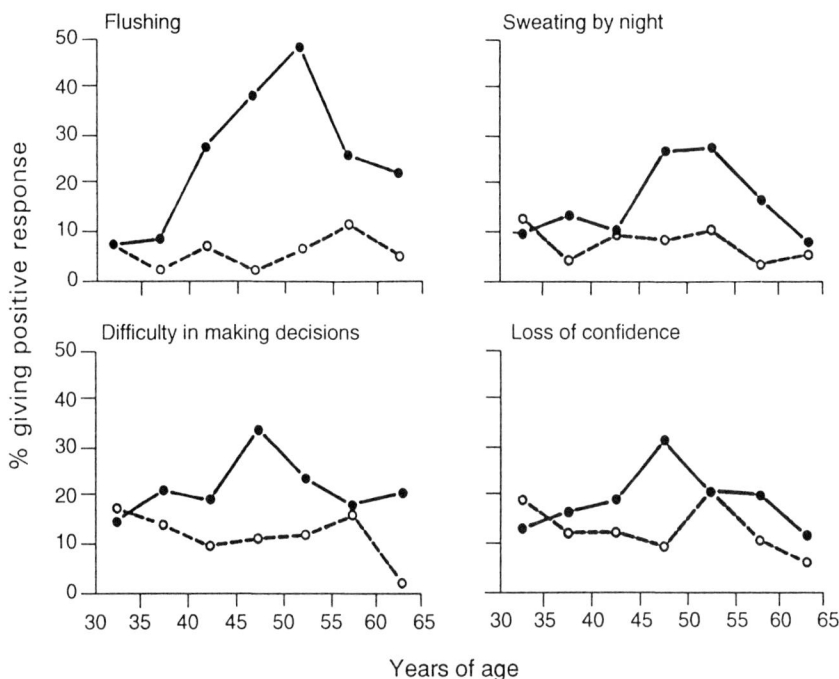

Figure 1 Percentage of men (o) and women (●) reporting the presence of various symptoms from age 30 years to age 65 years. From Bungay *et al.*[9] with permission

sweats may occur, which have similar features and physiological changes to those in women[7,8].

The association of other symptoms with the climacteric (Table 1) is less clear, but in an attempt to clarify the nature of the 'menopausal syndrome', Bungay and colleagues[9] carried out a postal questionnaire in a population sample of 1120 women and 510 men. Analysis of patterns of symptoms by age and sex showed that peaks of prevalence of flushes and sweats were closely associated with the mean age of the menopause, whereas less impressive peaks of prevalence of some minor mental symptoms were associated with an age just preceding the mean age of the menopause (Figure 1). The study provided no support for an association between the menopause and muscle and joint aches or headaches. However, they concluded that the 'menopausal syndrome' in women does exist.

An alternative way to try and assess which symptoms are associated with oestrogen deficiency is to note the response to oestrogen replacement therapy. Many studies in the earlier years of hormone replacement therapy (HRT) use reported apparent benefits of oestrogen, however, these studies were not adequately controlled. Subsequent reports have shown the large element of placebo response in women with menopausal symptoms, so only those which are double-blind placebo-controlled studies can identify the true effect of oestrogen. Confirmation of the superior benefit of oestrogen in reducing hot flushes was demonstrated by Coope and colleagues[10], with the placebo response being impressive up to 3 months, but the cross-over clearly showed the difference (Figure 2). Campbell and Whitehead[11] have demonstrated the effect of oestrogen on other symptoms in a double-blind cross-over study. Symptoms were quantified using a graphic rating scale to compare the effects of conjugated equine oestrogens and placebo (Figure 3). The oestrogen therapy was significantly more effective than placebo, not only in relieving hot flushes and sweats and vaginal dryness, but also in causing a significant reduction in insomnia, irritability, anxiety, urinary frequency, worry about self and age, and headaches, together with a significant improvement in memory, good spirits and optimism.

The reduction of flushes and sweats and the related disturbance of sleep results in an improvement in many other symptoms due to a 'domino effect'[11]. Women with severe menopausal symptoms but no flushes had similar benefits with oestrogen therapy although they had no change in insomnia, indicating that this is related to the vasomotor symptoms.

With longer duration of therapy (6 months cross-over) the highly significant placebo effect on vaginal dryness and urinary frequency disappeared. However, the significant placebo effect on a youthful skin appearance was maintained, together with a significant increase in skin greasiness. These results clearly demonstrate how confusing the placebo response can be and that patient assessment of skin texture and appearance in particular should not be used in the evaluation of oestrogen therapy. With the longer duration of therapy, the number of symptoms which were improved significantly compared

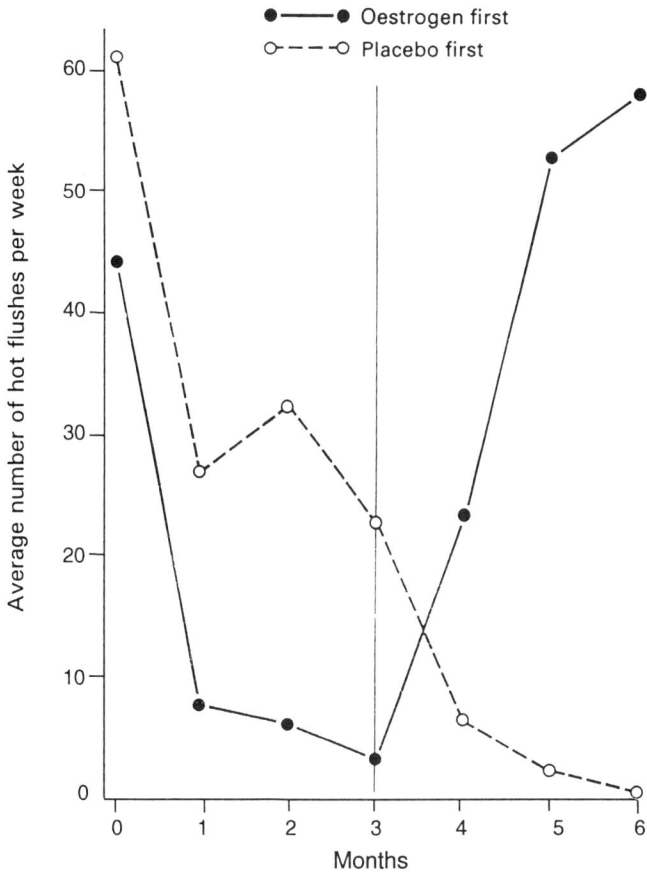

Figure 2 Hot flush count during a 6-month cross-over trial with Premarin 1.25 mg. Alteration in number of flushes per week after each month of therapy. From Coope *et al.*[10] with permission

to placebo was much reduced such that the truly oestrogen deficient symptoms may only be:

(1) Hot flushes;
(2) Vaginal dryness;
(3) Insomnia;
(4) Urinary frequency;
(5) Poor memory.

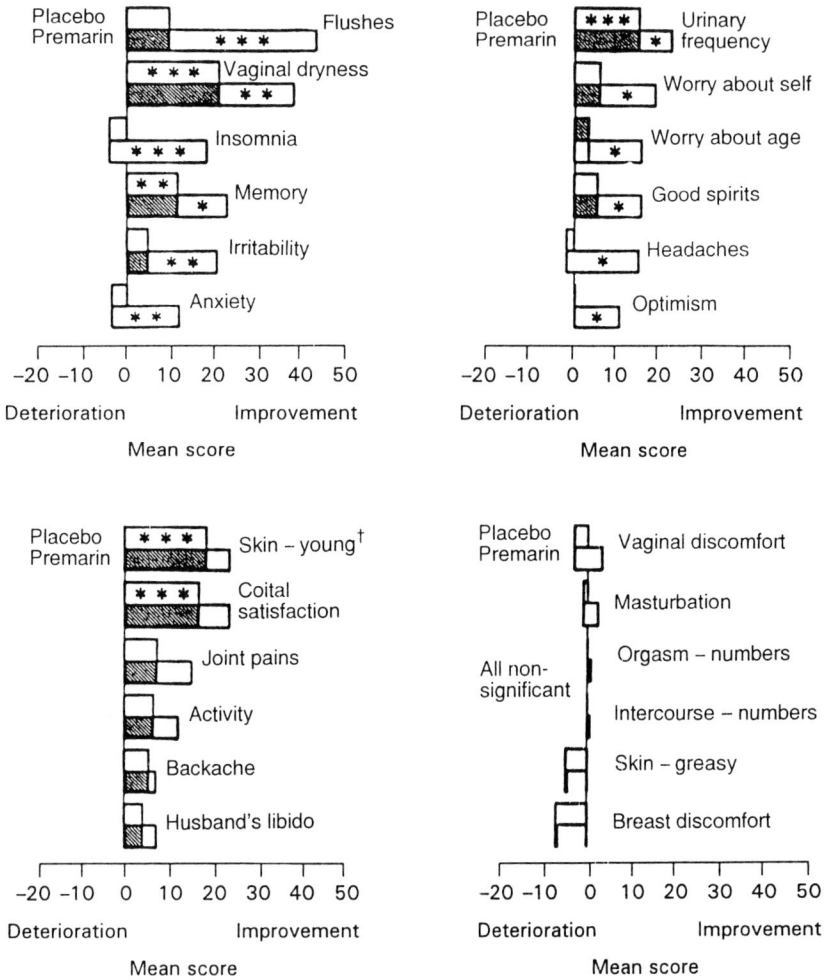

Figure 3 Differences in graphic rating scale scores for Premarin and placebo therapy in a 4-month study. [†]Significantly better on first course of treatment whether this was Premarin or placebo; * $p<0.05$; ** $p<0.01$; *** $p<0.001$. From Campbell and Whitehead[11] with permission

It is commonly thought that depression is more common in the climacteric, but the term has now been used to cover such a wide variation of symptoms and degrees of illness. A depressed mood is a normal human emotion that everyone experiences at some time, and feelings of sadness and disappointment are part of normal life experience. During the ovarian cycle variations in mood are common and premenstrual dysphoria is a component of the premenstrual syndrome. In the puerperium the increased risk of affective illness has also been attributed to rapid changes in circulating steroid hormone levels, but a specific psychological syndrome linked to the menopause has not been confirmed[12]. Women are two to three times more likely to report symptoms of depression than men at all ages, but there is no clear evidence that this increases at the menopause or that there is a peak of psychological morbidity[13]. Improvements in some psychological symptoms with oestrogen therapy may be due to a mental tonic effect of oestrogen[14].

Loss of libido is a non-specific term used frequently in publications on the menopause to indicate loss of sexual desire, which may be reported by about 45% of postmenopausal women[15]. Various physical factors related to ageing in both men and women will affect both desire and performance, but vaginal dryness and atrophic changes are specifically due to lack of oestrogen. Oestrogen therapy will improve this but if the libido does not respond, the addition of testosterone by subcutaneous pellet implant can be effective[16]. This benefit, however, has not been confirmed by others[17].

The symptoms discussed so far are generally associated with the perimenopause and early postmenopausal years. Oestrogen deficiency also contributes to ageing of the urogenital tract and various local symptoms which can cause particular distress in the older postmenopausal women[18]. Oestrogen receptors are present in the vagina, urethra, bladder and pelvic floor. Symptomatic, cytological and urodynamic changes in the lower urinary tract have been demonstrated during the menstrual cycle, pregnancy and after the menopause[19]. The vaginal epithelium shows the most marked changes resulting in dryness, irritation, burning and dyspareunia, all of which can be improved by either local or systemic oestrogen therapy. The extent to which urinary symptoms are associated with the menopause, however, is much less clear. Reports from different countries on the prevalence of urinary incontinence show wide variations. In British women the prevalence of stress incontinence seems to reach a peak at the age of 50 years and declines thereafter[20], whereas incontinent elderly Swedish women relate the onset of their symptoms to their last menstrual period[21]. Of 228 women attending a London menopause clinic complaining of climacteric symptoms, stress incontinence was found in over 50% and symptoms of urge incontinence in 26%. However, despite a common finding of urinary symptoms and urodynamic abnormalities, there was no correlation with the timing of the menopause[22].

Studies of the response to oestrogen therapy have largely been disappointing and few have been adequately placebo-controlled. There is no convincing evidence of benefit for stress incontinence, but frequency, nocturia and urgency can be improved as well as a reduction in the incidence of recurrent urinary tract infections[23]. It would seem, therefore, that stress incontinence is unlikely to be a result of oestrogen deficiency, whereas urge incontinence and other irritative bladder symptoms may be related[19].

THE HOT FLUSH

The hot flush is recognized by the medical profession and lay public as the most characteristic manifestation of the climacteric, and the benefits of oestrogen replacement therapy are well validated. Nevertheless there are several situations which seem inconsistent with simple oestrogen deficiency as a cause.

Prepubertal girls have low circulating oestrogen levels but do not experience flushes, whereas they may occur in pregnancy when there are high levels of oestrogen[24]. Not all women passing through the climacteric have flushes, and there is no apparent difference in the oestrogen levels of these women compared with those who do flush[25,26]. Flushing women, however, show greater diurnal variation of plasma oestradiol[25] which suggests that the rate of change of the plasma oestrogen levels could be a trigger for the flushing mechanism, or that for each individual there is a range of oestrogen levels within which flushes will occur but above or below which they will not. Flushes are more prevalent and severe in women who experience acute oestrogen withdrawal, such as following bilateral oophorectomy, than in those experiencing the gradual ovarian failure of a natural climacteric. In addition, hot flushes are commonly the first symptom of the climacteric and do not usually persist into later postmenopausal years when circulating oestrogen levels are even lower.

Priming with oestrogen may be an essential prerequisite for flushing, as young women with ovarian dysgenesis do not have flushes unless they are given oestrogen replacement therapy which is stopped later. Furthermore, women taking clomiphene or tamoxifen therapy may also complain of flushes due to the anti-oestrogenic effect at the hypothalamus.

There is also no difference in overall circulating plasma levels of follicle stimulating hormone (FSH) and luteinizing hormone (LH) between postmenopausal women who flush and those who do not[25,26], but a temporal association of flushes with the pulsatile release of LH from the pituitary has been demonstrated[27] (Figure 4). However, elimination of these LH pulses by luteinizing hormone releasing hormone (LHRH) analogue does not affect the frequency of flushing, indicating that LH is merely associated with the flush rather than being causative[28,29]. Neuroendocrine events in the hypothalamus which govern the pulsatile release of LHRH may be linked functionally with thermoregulation, as some of the hypothalamic neurones that contain LHRH are in close proximity to the pre-optic nuclei that regulate body temperature[30]. Although, the exact mechanism of flushing is not known, it is generally considered that it is in part due to a disturbance of the thermoregulating centre.

The hot flush is different from other flushes associated with medical conditions such as the carcinoid or dumping syndromes, phaeochromocytoma and autonomic epilepsy, and from the common blush[31]. In most women the flush starts on the face, neck, head or chest and the initial focal point may be very specific such as an earlobe, forehead or between the breasts. Subsequent spread of the sensation of heat may be in any direction, and some feel it over the whole body.

Temperature changes during the flush vary from an increase of about 1°C on the face[32] to 5°C in the fingers and toes, whereas core temperature as recorded in the oesophagus, rectum, vagina and tympanic membrane falls due to the heat losing effect of peripheral vasodilatation[33,34]. Other characteristic features of the hot flush have been identified in studies of the physiological changes[35] (Figure 5). Increases of the heart rate and peripheral blood flow are accompan-

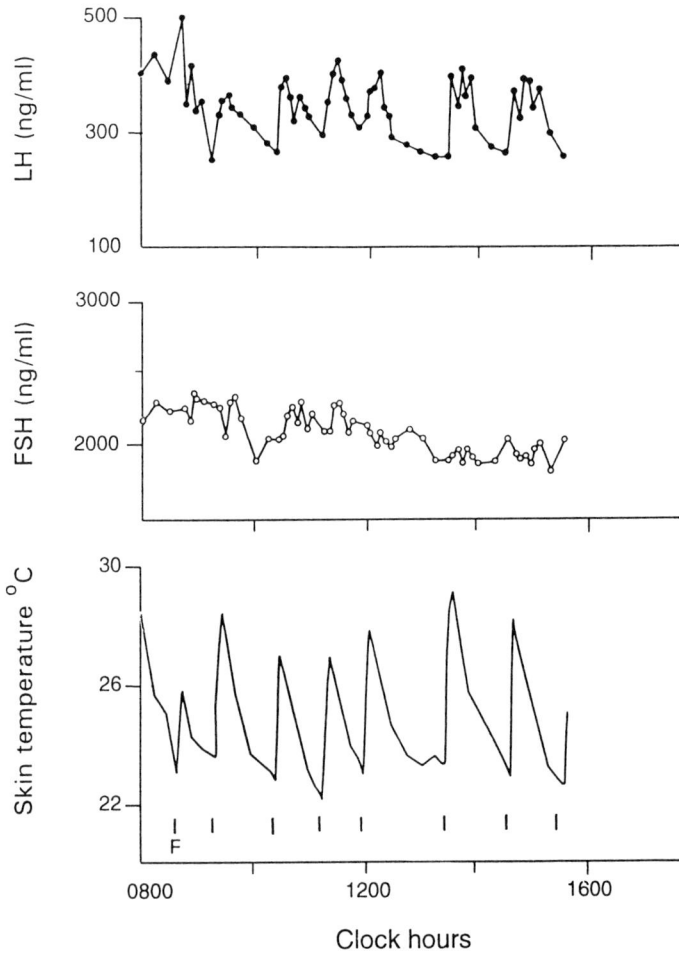

Figure 4 Changes in cutaneous finger temperature, serum luteinizing hormone (LH) and follicle stimulating hormone (FSH) levels during an 8-h study of a postmenopausal woman. From Tataryn *et al.*[27] with permission

ied by a dramatic fall in the galvanic skin resistance (reflected in Figure 5 by marked fluctuations of the baseline of the single lead electro-cardiograph (ECG) trace), which is a reflection of increased sympathetic drive. This is unique to the menopausal flush. In premenopausal women heat-induced peripheral vasodilatation is not accompanied by changes in heart rate, ECG baseline or skin resist-

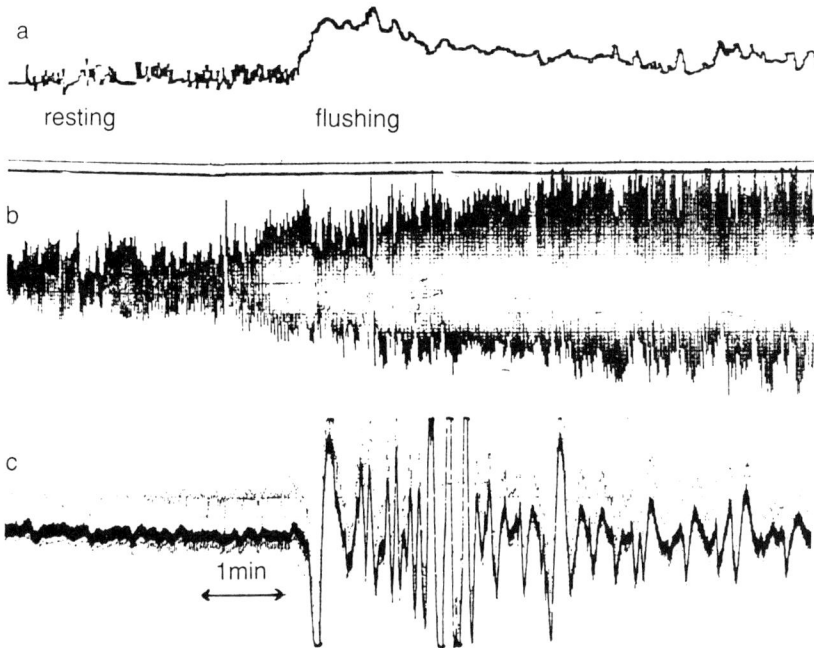

Figure 5 Physiological recordings of (a) heart rate beats/min, (b) digital plethysmograph and (c) electro-cardiograph (ECG) from a postmenopausal woman before and during a hot flush. From Sturdee *et al.*[35] with permission

ance, so the pronounced changes in these parameters with hot flushes are not a result of vasodilatation or sweating. A temporary increase in sympathetic drive followed by local release of a vasodilator factor in the peripheral vessel wall might explain these events[31].

CONCLUSIONS

The climacteric and postmenopausal years can produce a wide spectrum of symptomatic responses from minimal change to dramatic effects on the quality of life. Not all are due directly to lack of oestrogen and the individual response to this time of life may be influenced by many other factors. Oestrogen therapy can be very beneficial due to a direct effect of the hormone, as well as a mental tonic effect and a substantial although short-lived placebo response.

REFERENCES

1. McKinlay, S.M. and Jeffreys, M. (1974). The menopausal syndrome. *Br. J. Prevent. Soc. Med.*, **28**, 108–15
2. Medical Women's Federation (1933). An investigation of the menopause in one thousand women. *Lancet*, **1**, 106–8
3. Hammar, M., Berg, G., Fahraeus, L. and Larsson-Cohn, U. (1984). Climacteric symptoms in an unselected sample of Swedish women. *Maturitas*, **6**, 345–50
4. Lock, M. (1991). Hot flushes in cultural context: the Japanese case as a cautionary tale for the West. In Schönbaum, E. (ed.) *The Climacteric Hot Flush. Prog. Basic Clin. Pharmacol.* Vol. 6, pp. 40–60. (Basel: Karger)
5. McLaren, H.C. (1941). The induced menopause. *J. Obstet. Gynaecol. Br. Emp.*, **48**, 23–40
6. Chakravarti, S., Collins, W.P., Newton, J.R., Oram, D.H. and Studd, J.W.W. (1977). Endocrine changes and symptomatology after oophorectomy in premenopausal women. *Br. J. Obstet. Gynaecol.*, **84**, 769–75
7. Feldman, J.M., Postlethwaite, R.W. and Glenn, J.F. (1976). Hot flushes and sweats in men with testicular insufficiency. *Arch. Intern. Med.*, **136**, 606–8
8. Ginsburg, J. and O'Reilly, B. (1983). Climacteric flushing in a man. *Br. Med. J.*, **287**, 262
9. Bungay, G.T., Vessey, M.P. and McPherson, C.K. (1980). Study of symptoms in middle life with special reference to the menopause. *Br. Med. J.*, **2**, 181–3
10. Coope, J., Thomson, J.M. and Poller, L. (1975). Effects of 'natural oestrogen' replacement therapy on menopausal symptoms and blood clotting. *Br. Med. J.*, **4**, 139–43
11. Campbell, S. and Whitehead, M.I. (1977). Oestrogen therapy and the menopausal syndrome. In Greenblatt, R.B. and Studd, J.W.W. (eds.) *The Menopause. Clinics in Obstetrics and Gynaecology*, **4** (1), pp. 31–47. (London, Philadelphia, Toronto: W.B. Saunders Co. Ltd.)
12. Appleby, L., Montgomery, J. and Studd, J.W.W. (1991). Oestrogens and affective disorders. In Studd, J. (ed.) *Progress in Obstetrics and Gynaecology*, Vol. 9, pp. 289–302. (London: Churchill Livingstone)
13. Ballinger, C.B. (1975). Psychiatric morbidity and the menopause; screening of a general population sample. *Br. Med. J.*, **2**, 344–6
14. Utian, W.H. (1972). The mental tonic effect of oestrogens administered to oophorectomised females. *S. Afr. Med. J.*, **46**, 1079–82
15. Sarrel, P. and Whitehead, M.I. (1985). Sex and menopause: defining the issues. *Maturitas*, **7**, 217–24

16. Brincat, M., Magos, A.L. and Studd, J.W.W. (1984). Subcutaneous hormone implants for the control of climacteric symptoms: a prospective study. *Lancet*, **1**, 16–18

17. Dow, M.G.T., Hart, D.M. and Forrest, C.A. (1983). Hormonal treatment of sexual unresponsiveness in postmenopausal women: a comparative study. *Br. J. Obstet. Gynaecol.*, **90**, 361–6

18. Barlow, D.H., Cardozo, L.D., Francis, R.M., Griffin, M., Hart, D.M., Stephens, E. and Sturdee, D.W. (1996). Urogenital ageing and its effect on sexual health in older British women. *Br. J. Obstet. Gynaecol.*, in press

19. Cardozo, L.D. and Kelleher, C.J. (1995). Sex hormones, the menopause and urinary problems. *Gynecol. Endocrinol.*, **9**, 75–84

20. Jolleys, J.V. (1988). Reported prevalence of urinary incontinence in women in general practice. *Br. Med. J.*, **296**, 1300–2

21. Iosif, C.S. and Bekassy, Z. (1984). Prevalence of genito-urinary symptoms in the later menopause. *Acta Obstet. Gynecol. Scand.*, **63**, 257–60

22. Versi, E. and Cardozo, L.D. (1988). Oestrogens and lower urinary tract function. In Studd, J.W.W. and Whitehead, M.I. (eds.) *The Menopause*, pp.76–84. (Oxford: Blackwell Scientific Publications)

23. Raz, R. and Stamm, W.E. (1993). A controlled trial of intravaginal estriol in postmenopausal women with recurrent urinary tract infections. *N. Engl. J. Med.*, **329**, 753–6

24. Ginsburg, J. and Duncan, S.L.B. (1967). Peripheral blood flow in normal pregnancy. *Cardiovas. Res.*, **1**, 132–7

25. Campbell, S., Breeson, A.J., Kitchin, Y., Fergusson, I.K. and Biswas, S. (1976). Intensive steroid and protein hormone profiles on post-menopausal women experiencing hot flushes and a group of controls. In Campbell, S. (ed.) *The Management of the Menopause and Post-Menopausal Years*, pp. 63–77. (Lancaster: MTP Press Ltd.)

26. Hutton, J.D., Jacobs, H.S., Murray, M.A.F. and James, V.H.T. (1978). Relationship between plasma oestrone and oestradiol and climacteric symptoms. *Lancet*, **1**, 678–81

27. Tataryn, I.V., Meldrum, D.R., Lu, K. H., Frumar, A.M. and Judd, H.L. (1979). LH, FSH and skin temperature during the menopausal hot flushes. *J. Clin. Endocrinol. Metab.*, **49**, 152–4

28. Lightman, S.L., Jacobs, H.S. and Maguire, A.K. (1982). Down regulation of gonadotrophic secretion in postmenopausal women by a superactive LHRH analogue: lack of effect on menopausal flushing. *Br. J. Obstet. Gynaecol.*, **89**, 977–80

29. Shaw, R.W., Kerr-Wilson, R.H.J., Fraser, H.M., McNeilly, A.S., Howie, P.W. and Sandow, J. (1985). Effect of an intranasal LHRH agonist on

gonadotrophins and hot flushes in post-menopausal women. *Maturitas*, **7**, 161–7

30. Simpkins, J.W. and Kalra, S.P. (1979). Central site(s) of norepinephrine and LHRH interaction. *Fed. Proc.*, **38**, 1107

31. Sturdee, D.W. and Brincat, M. (1988). The hot flush. In Studd, J.W.W. and Whitehead, M.I. (eds.) *The Menopause*, pp. 24–42. (Oxford: Blackwell Scientific Publications)

32. Sturdee, D.W. and Reece, B.L. (1979). Thermography of menopausal hot flushes. *Maturitas*, **1**, 201–5

33. Molnar, G.W. (1975). Body temperatures during menopausal hot flushes. *J. Appl. Physiol.*, **38**, 499–501

34. Kronenberg, F., Cote, L.J., Linkie, D.M., Dyrenfurther, I. and Downey, J.A. (1984). Menopausal hot flushes: thermoregulatory, cardiovascular and circulating catecholamines and LH changes. *Maturitas*, **6**, 31–43

35. Sturdee, D.W., Wilson, K.A., Pipili, E. and Crocker, A.D. (1978). Physiological aspects of menopausal hot flush. *Br. Med. J.*, **2**, 79–80

2

Lipid changes and cardiovascular implications

J.C. Stevenson

INTRODUCTION

Cardiovascular disease is the major cause of death in women just as it is in men, but because these deaths occur at a later age than in men the importance of the disease in women is often overlooked. The incidence of cardiovascular disease, particularly coronary heart disease (CHD), increases with age in women as well as in men, but in women there is an additional increase due to the menopause[1]. Indeed, women may have a 3.4-fold greater risk of atherosclerosis after a natural menopause[2]. It has long been recognized that premature menopause, whether natural[3] or surgical[4], results in premature CHD.

LIPIDS, LIPOPROTEINS AND CARDIOVASCULAR DISEASE

It is well established that high circulating levels of cholesterol are associated with increased incidence of CHD. Low density lipoproteins (LDL) account for the major portion of total plasma cholesterol in most individuals, and increased levels of LDL cholesterol lead to increased risk of CHD whilst lowering the levels reduces the risk[5]. The clearance of LDL and the intermediate density lipoproteins (IDL) is effected by hepatic receptors but this process is slow and operates at near saturation of the receptors[6]. Thus with high LDL concentrations, their relatively long half-life in the circulation makes them more susceptible to modification or damage and more likely to be retained intramurally in the arteries. Postprandial lipoprotein remnants are also atherogenic and thus the efficiency of remnant clearance is important.

LDL comprises various subclasses differing in size, chemical composition and density[7]. Lipoprotein (a) is an LDL which contains apolipoprotein B and apolipoprotein (a), the latter being structurally a giant mutant of plasminogen[8] (for review, see[9]). Lipoprotein (a) appears to be an independent lipoprotein risk marker for CHD, with high levels being associated with increased risk for CHD, but probably only when LDL levels are also raised. Lipoprotein (a) is atherogenic largely because of its propensity for retention in the arterial wall. It binds avidly to arterial proteoglycans[10], and also enhances arterial LDL retention[11]. Lipoprotein (a) is also potentially thrombogenic because of its structural homology with plasminogen. Thus, it may compete with plasminogen for binding sites and inhibit fibrinolysis, and it also binds fibrin[12].

The size of LDL particles vary and can be classified into subgroups accordingly. It has been shown that LDL particle size is clinically important, with patients with CHD and particularly female patients having an increased proportion of small dense LDL compared with healthy controls[13], a pattern described as subtype B. These small dense LDL particles are more atherogenic, perhaps because they are more readily cleared through scavenger mechanisms rather than by the $apoB_{100}$ receptors, and also because they may be more susceptible to oxidative damage[14]. Small dense LDL are found in individuals with raised triglycerides and low HDL[13] and are a feature of the insulin resistance syndrome[15].

High density lipoproteins (HDL) may participate in reverse cholesterol transport whereby they remove cholesterol from tissues and return it to the liver for excretion or resecretion. Thus, HDL levels are inversely associated with CHD risk[16], with high levels considered to be protective. The HDL_2 subfraction is considered to be the subfraction which confers the most benefit, and HDL_2 can be catabolized by hepatic lipase. Thus, adiposity and androgens, both of which increase hepatic lipase activity, are associated with low HDL_2

levels. Triglyceride levels are inversely associated with HDL and HDL$_2$ levels[17]. Increased hepatic triglyceride production leads to increased levels of triglyceride-rich very low density lipoproteins (VLDL). Reduced VLDL clearance results in increased plasma residence of VLDL remnants, decreased HDL$_2$ and increased IDL levels[6], an atherogenic lipoprotein profile. Thus low levels of HDL and HDL$_2$ may reflect a reduction in reverse cholesterol transport or a reduction in VLDL remnant clearance, and it is not clear which is more important.

LIPOPROTEINS AND THE DEVELOPMENT OF ATHEROMA

Several processes have been implicated in the initiation of atheromatous lesions, including endothelial injury or increased permeability, and turbulent blood flow causing sheer stress-induced endothelial alteration. Recently, a unifying hypothesis for the initial development of the atherosclerotic lesion has been advanced[18]. This hypothesis proposes that the initial and most important event is the subendothelial retention of atherogenic lipoproteins, and that arterial proteoglycans, together with lipoprotein lipase and sphingomyelinase, are largely responsible for intramural retention of LDL and particularly lipoprotein (a). These retained lipoproteins have increased sensitivity to oxidation. Oxidized lipoproteins are chemo-attractive to monocytes, smooth muscle cells and T-lymphocytes, and are avidly taken up to form foam cells which then progress to the development of the atheromatous plaque. Alterations in endothelial permeability, as seen in smoking and dyslipidaemias, may contribute to this process, and sheer stress from turbulent blood flow may induce lipoprotein retention through stimulating proteoglycan synthesis. However, the factors responsible for focal lipoprotein retention and subsequent lesion development are still largely unknown.

EFFECTS OF MENOPAUSE ON LIPIDS AND LIPOPROTEINS

Whilst profound effects of exogenous sex steroids on lipids and lipoproteins have been demonstrated, there has been more controversy as to the effects of endogenous female hormones. This is partly due to the fact that age and menopause are closely related, and many cross-sectional studies did not include sufficient numbers or a wide enough age range to permit the age adjustments necessary to determine effects of the menopause. Furthermore, menopausal status had often not been adequately determined. Studies of pre- and postmenopausal women around the age of the menopause will inevitably be confounded by the inclusion of perimenopausal women of similar hormonal status in both groups. The use of women with premature menopause who can be matched with premenopausal controls may be invalid as the former are not representative of the normal population. Equally, studies of women undergoing surgical menopause can be confounded by the effects of the surgery itself.

In a large cross-sectional study of 542 healthy non-obese Caucasian females aged between 18 and 70 years, we measured lipids and lipoproteins[17]. Premenopausal status was defined by a regular menstrual cycle whilst postmenopausal status was defined by amenorrhoea and elevated gonadotrophins. In order to study the effects of the menopause independently of age, multiple linear regression analyses were performed separately for the premenopausal and postmenopausal women and these were used to standardize for confounding variables, such as chronological age, and anthropometric and lifestyle parameters. The results are summarized in Figure 1. The standardized mean values for total cholesterol and triglycerides, LDL and HDL_3 cholesterol were significantly higher in postmenopausal women whilst those of HDL and particularly HDL_2 cholesterol were significantly lower. Our findings are in agreement with longitudinal studies[19,20]. A further analysis of one of these studies[21] demonstrated the striking effect of the menopause on HDL_2 cholesterol, in accordance with our findings. These various changes in lipids and lipoproteins should be regarded as potentially detrimental in terms of CHD risk.

Other adverse changes include a reported increase in lipoprotein (a)[22] and a shift in LDL particle size towards smaller denser LDL[23].

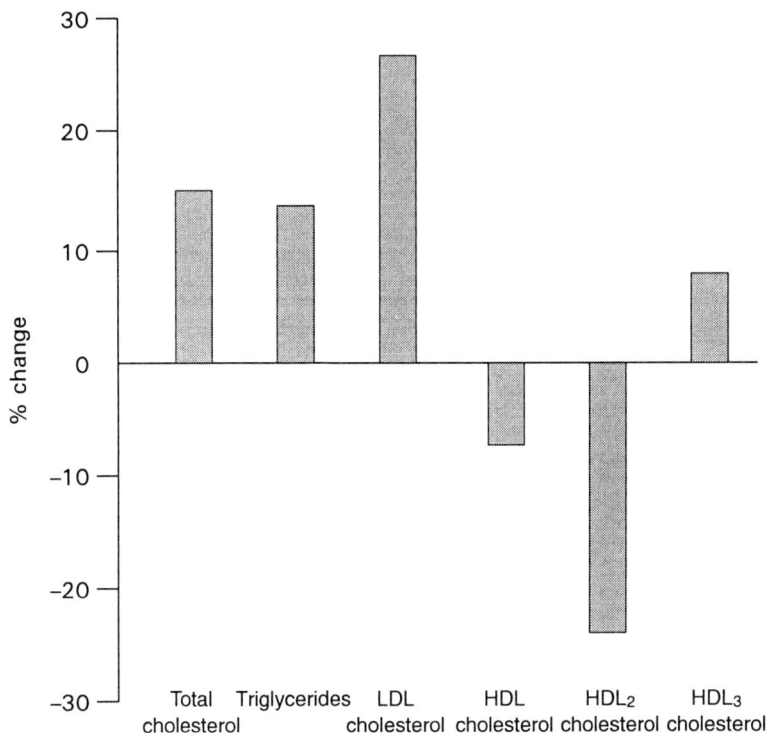

Figure 1 Changes in serum lipids and lipoproteins resulting from the meno-pause. Modified from Stevenson *et al.*[17]

EFFECTS OF HRT ON LIPIDS AND LIPOPROTEINS

The effects of HRT on lipids and lipoproteins will depend on the particular oestrogen given, its dose and its route of administration. These effects may be modified if a progestogen is added as part of the HRT, again depending on the particular steroid used and its route of administration. Such progestogen effects may also depend on the regimen employed, so that the effects may be more pro-nounced if the progestogen is given in a continuous rather than a cyclical fashion.

It is well established that oestrogen lowers total cholesterol, irrespec-tive of type of steroid or route of administration, and this effect is main-

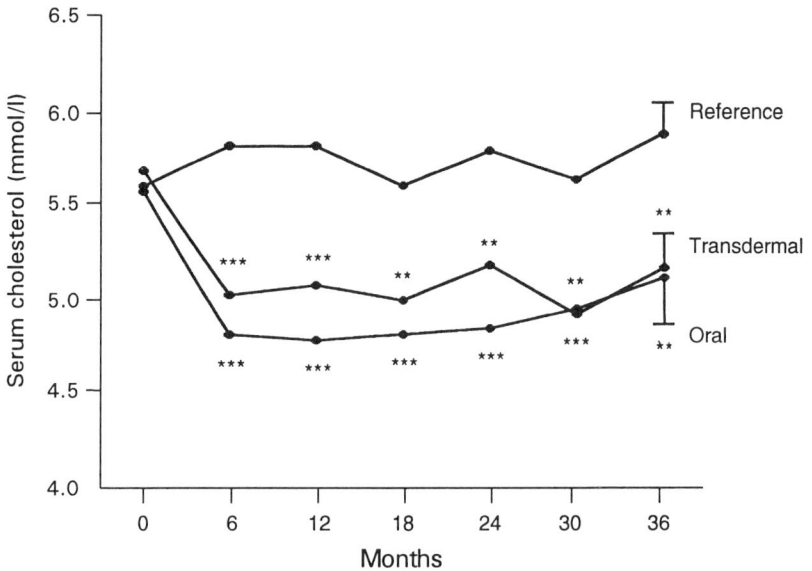

Figure 2 Long-term changes in serum cholesterol concentrations in post-menopausal women receiving no treatment (reference), transdermal oestradiol 17β 0.05 mg daily with cyclic norethisterone acetate 0.15 mg (transdermal), or oral conjugated equine oestrogens 0.625 mg daily with cyclic norgestrel 0.15 mg (oral) **$p < 0.01$; ***$p < 0.001$. From Whitcroft *et al.*[24] with permission

tained in the long-term whilst on treatment[24] (Figure 2). This lowering of cholesterol results primarily from a decrease in LDL cholesterol concentrations due to an up-regulation of $apoB_{100}$ receptors. The greatest magnitude of decrease in LDL with HRT appears to be seen in those with the highest baseline levels[25]. Oestrogen may reduce the levels of lipoprotein (a), although such an effect appears rather small and has not been extensively studied. Qualitative changes in LDL induced by HRT may also be of relevance. HRT appears to increase the proportion of small dense LDL particles[26]. However. some studies have suggested that HRT in fact decreases the proportion of larger LDL particles[27], and particularly IDL cholesterol[28], thus this change in LDL subtype pattern is not necessarily adverse. Oestrogen appears to protect against lipoprotein oxidation, thereby rendering the LDL less atherogenic[29], and also improves the postprandial clearance of potentially atherogenic lipoprotein remnants[28].

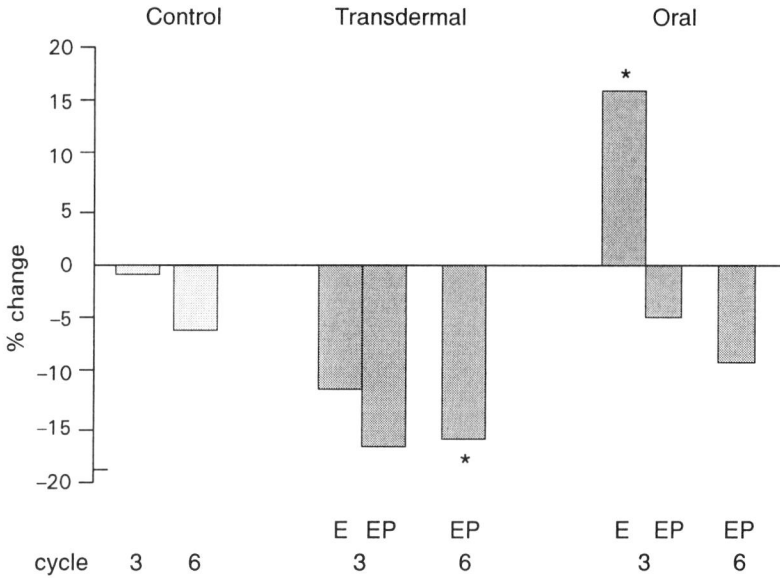

Figure 3 Changes in triglyceride concentrations in postmenopausal women receiving no treatment (control), transdermal oestradiol 17β 0.05 mg daily with cyclic norethisterone acetate 0.15 mg (transdermal), or oral conjugated equine oestrogens 0.625 mg daily with cyclic norgestrel 0.15 mg (oral). *$p < 0.05$. From Crook *et al*.[30] with permission

Orally administered oestrogen increases HDL cholesterol, and particularly the HDL_2 subfraction which is thought to confer a protective effect against atherosclerosis development, by inhibiting hepatic lipase activity and by increasing the hepatic synthesis of apolipoprotein A-I. Transdermal oestradiol appears to have a less marked effect on HDL cholesterol[30].

The type and route of administration of oestrogen determines its effects on triglycerides. As triglycerides appear to be a particular risk factor for CHD in women[31], this is of potential importance. Conjugated equine oestrogens cause an increase in triglycerides[30], an effect which is pharmacological, resulting from the hepatic first-pass effect of this steroid. Orally administered oestradiol has little or no effect on raising triglycerides, but transdermal oestradiol causes a reduction in triglycerides[30] which is the physiological effect of oestrogen (Figure 3).

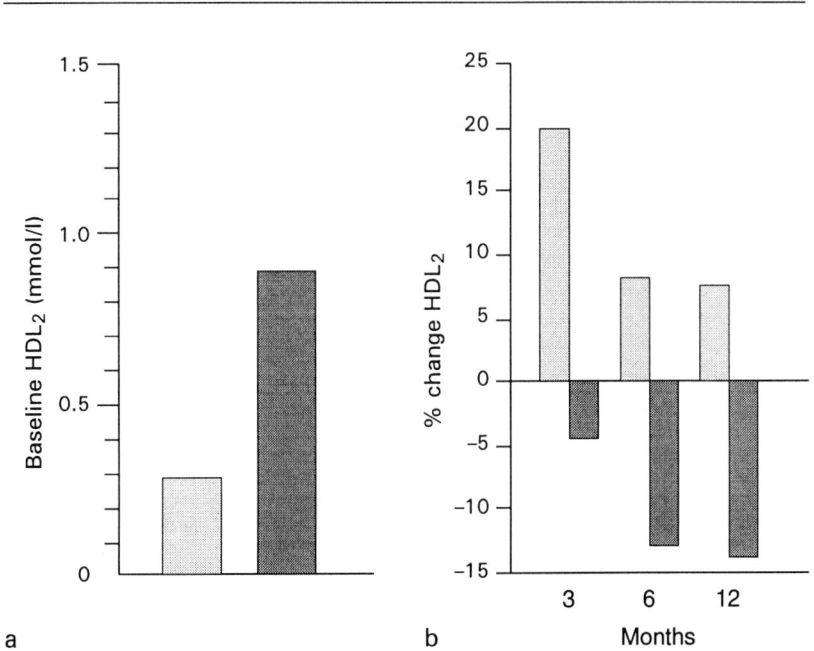

Figure 4 Postmenopausal women selected according to high (dark bars) or low (light bars) baseline HDL$_2$ cholesterol level (a) and their subsequent response to oral and transdermal HRT during the oestrogen alone phase of treatment at 3 months, and during the combined oestrogen/progestogen phases at 6 and 12 months (b). From Whitcroft *et al.*[24] and Crook *et al.*[30] with permission

Progestogens have differing effects on lipids and lipoproteins, depending more on their androgenicity and perhaps dose duration rather than their route of administration. The addition of progestogens to oestrogen therapy has no obvious adverse effect in terms of lowering of LDL, since they increase LDL production but also increase their clearance[32]. Progestogens which are derived from testosterone, such as norgestrel, reverse the HDL-raising effect of oestrogen[30] because they increase hepatic lipase activity. This effect is regarded as potentially disadvantageous, although it is most pronounced in patients with high HDL$_2$ levels and paradoxically may not occur in those with low HDL$_2$ levels[33] (Figure 4). Thus, in analogy to the effects of HRT on LDL, patients with the greatest dispersions from normal in HDL$_2$ concentrations may show the most

22

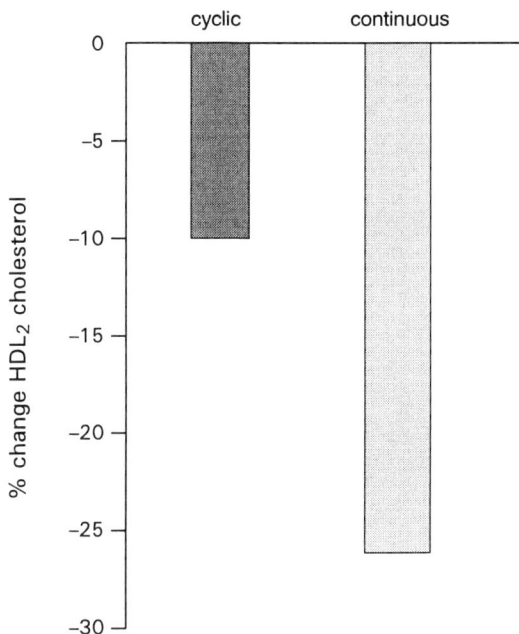

Figure 5 Comparison of HDL$_2$ cholesterol changes in the combined phase of treatment in postmenopausal women receiving either continuous conjugated equine oestrogens 0.625 mg daily and cyclic *dl*-norgestrel 0.15 mg daily (dark bar) or continuous combined oestradiol 17β 1 mg daily and desogestrel 0.15 mg daily (light bar). From Crook *et al.*[30] and Marsh *et al.*[36]

beneficial response in changes seen with HRT. Furthermore, it is not known whether the reduction in HDL reflects any impairment in remnant clearance and thus the clinical significance of lowering HDL remains to be determined. In contrast, the less androgenic progestogens do not impede the oestrogen-induced increase in HDL cholesterol to any great extent. Furthermore, androgenic steroids lower lipoprotein (a)[34–36], an effect which might be beneficial. Any effect on lipoprotein oxidation is currently unknown.

Depending on their androgenicity, progestogens reduce VLDL secretion and this results in a lowering of triglycerides[30], an effect which is clearly beneficial. Such an effect is not seen with the non-androgenic progestogens. The duration of progestogen administration in HRT may also be important. For example, desogestrel is a progestogen derived from norgestrel and has less androgenic effects than the parent molecule. However, continuous administration of desogestrel together with oestradiol results in a lowering of HDL_2 by 26%[36] compared with a reduction of only 10% during the combined phase of continuous conjugated equine oestrogens but cyclical norgestrel[30] (Figure 5).

It is thus possible to obtain a variety of different effects on lipids and lipoproteins with HRT, depending on the choice of steroids used and their route of administration. Overall, the effects of most HRT on lipids and lipoproteins would seem to be in balance beneficial, and of course there are many other factors which influence cardiovascular risk that are also beneficially affected by HRT[37]. Nevertheless, future HRT regimens should ideally be tailored to produce the most favourable lipid and lipoprotein pattern, particularly in the case of the regimens which attempt to avoid cyclical bleeding.

ACKNOWLEDGEMENTS

I am grateful for the support of the Heart Disease and Diabetes Research Trust, and the Cecil Rosen Foundation.

REFERENCES

1. Gordon, T., Kannel, W.B., Hjortland, M.C. and McNamara, P.M. (1978). Menopause and coronary heart disease. The Framingham Study. *Ann. Intern. Med.*, **89**, 157–61
2. Wittemen, J., Grobbee, D., Kok, F., Hofman, A. and Valkenburg, H. (1989). Increased risk of atherosclerosis in women after the menopause. *Br. Med. J.*, **298**, 642–4
3. Sznajderman, M. and Oliver, M.F. (1963). Spontaneous premature menopause, ischaemic heart disease and serum lipids. *Lancet*, **1**, 962–4
4. Oliver, M.F. and Boyd, G.S. (1959). Effect of bilateral ovariectomy on coronary artery disease and serum lipid levels. *Lancet*, **2**, 690–2
5. Scandinavian Simvastatin Survival Study Group (1994). Randomised trial of cholesterol lowering in 4444 patients with coronary heart disease: the Scandinavian Simvastatin Survival Study (4S). *Lancet*, **344**, 1383–9

6. Krauss, R.M. (1991). The tangled web of coronary risk factors. *Am. J. Med.*, **90** (Suppl. 2A), 36S–41S

7. Shen, M.M.S., Krauss, R.M., Lindgren, F.T. and Forte, T.M. (1981). Heterogeneity of serum low density lipoproteins in normal human subjects. *J. Lipid Res.*, **22**, 236–44

8. Utermann, G. (1989). The mysteries of lipoprotein (a). *Science*, **264**, 904–10

9. Maher, V. M. G. and Brown, B.G. (1995). Lipoprotein (a) and coronary heart disease. *Curr. Opin. Lipidol.*, **6**, 229–35

10. Dahlén, G., Ericson, C. and Berg, K. (1978). In vitro studies of the interaction of isolated Lp(a) lipoprotein and other serum lipoproteins with glycosaminoglycans. *Clin. Genet.*, **14**, 36–42

11. Yashiro, A., O'Neil, J. and Hoff, H.F. (1993). Insoluble complex formation of lipoprotein (a) with low density lipoprotein in the presence of calcium ions. *J. Biol. Chem.*, **268**, 4709–15

12. Loscalzo, J., Weinfeld, M., Fless, G.M. and Scanu, A.M. (1990). Lipoprotein (a), fibrin binding and plasminogen activation. *Arteriosclerosis*, **10**, 240–5

13. Austin, M.A., Breslow, J.L., Hennekens, C.H., Buring, J.E., Willett, W.C. and Krauss, R.M. (1988). Low density lipoprotein subclass patterns and risk of myocardial infarction. *J. Am. Med. Assoc.*, **26**, 1917–21

14. Tribble, D.L., Holl, L.G., Wood, P.D. and Krauss, R.M. (1992). Variations in oxidative susceptibility among six low density lipoprotein subfractions of differing density and particle size. *Atherosclerosis*, **93**, 189–99

15. Reaven, G.M., Ida Chen, Y.-D., Jeppesen, J., Maheux, P. and Krauss, R.M. (1993). Insulin resistance and hyperinsulinaemia in individuals with small dense low density lipoprotein particles. *J. Clin. Invest.*, **92**, 141–6

16. Miller, N.E. (1987). Associations of high-density lipoprotein subclasses and apolipoproteins with ischaemic heart disease and coronary atherosclerosis. *Am. Heart J.*, **113**, 589–97

17. Stevenson, J.C., Crook, D. and Godsland, I.F. (1993). Influence of age and menopause on serum lipids and lipoproteins in healthy women. *Atherosclerosis*, **98**, 83–90

18. Williams, K.J. and Tabas, I. (1995). The response-to-retention hypothesis of early atherogenesis. *Arterioscler. Thromb.*, **15**, 551–61

19. Jensen, J., Nilas, L. and Christiansen, C. (1990). Influence of menopause on serum lipids and lipoproteins. *Maturitas*, **12**, 321–31

20. Matthews, K.A., Meilahn, E., Kuller, L.H., Helsey, S.F., Caggiula, A.W. and Wing, R.R. (1989). Menopause and risk factors for coronary heart disease. *N. Engl. J. Med.*, **321**, 641–46

21. Kuller, L.H., Gutai, J.P., Meilahn, E., Matthews, K.A. and Plantinga, P. (1990). Relationship of endogenous sex steroid hormones to lipids and apoproteins in postmenopausal women. *Arteriosclerosis*, **10**, 1058–60

22. Meilahn, E.N., Kuller, L.H., Matthews, K.A. and Stein, A. (1991). Lp(a) concentrations among pre- and postmenopausal women over time: the Healthy Women Study. *Circulation*, **84** (Suppl. II), 546

23. Campos, H., McNamara, J.R., Wilson, P.W.F., Ordovas, J.M. and Schaefer, E.J. (1988). Differences in low density lipoprotein subfractions and apolipoproteins in premenopausal and postmenopausal women. *J. Clin. Endocrinol. Metab.*, **67**, 30–5

24. Whitcroft, S.I., Crook, D., Marsh, M.S., Ellerington, M.C., Whitehead, M.I. and Stevenson, J.C. (1994). Long-term effects of oral and transdermal hormone replacement therapies on serum lipid and lipoprotein concentrations. *Obstet. Gynecol.*, **84**, 222–6

25. Tikkanen, M.J., Kuusi, T., Vartiainen, E. and Nikkila, E.A. (1979). Treatment of postmenopausal hypercholesterolaemia with oestradiol. *Acta Obstet. Gynecol.*, **88** (Suppl.), 83–8

26. van der Mooren, M.J., de Graaf, J., Demacker, P.N., de Haan, A.F. and Rolland, R. (1994). Changes in the low-density lipoprotein profile during 17beta-oestradiol-dydrogesterone therapy in postmenopausal women. *Metabolism*, **43**, 799–802

27. Campos, H., Sacks, F.M., Walsh, B.W., Schiff, I., O'Hanesian, M.A. and Krauss, R.M. (1993). Differential aspects of estrogen on low-density lipoprotein subclasses in healthy postmenopausal women. *Metabolism*, **42**, 1153–8

28. Westerveld, H.T., Kock, L.A.W., van Rijn, J.M., Erkelens, D.W. and de Bruin, T.W.A. (1995). 17β-estradiol improves postprandial lipid metabolism in postmenopausal women. *J. Clin. Endocrinol. Metab.*, **80**, 249–53

29. Sack, M.N., Rader, D.J. and Cannon, R.O. (1994). Oestrogen and inhibition of oxidation of low-density lipoproteins in postmenopausal women. *Lancet*, **343**, 269–70

30. Crook, D., Cust, M.P., Gangar, K.F., Worthington, M., Hillard, T.C., Stevenson, J.C., Whitehead, M.I. and Wynn, V. (1992). Comparison of transdermal and oral estrogen/progestin hormone replacement therapy: effects on serum lipids and lipoproteins. *Am. J. Obstet. Gynecol.*, **166**, 950–5

31. Bengtsson, C., Björkelund, C., Lapidus, L. and Lissner, L. (1993). Associations of serum lipid concentrations and obesity with mortality in women: 20 year follow up of participants in prospective population study in Gothenburg, Sweden. *Br. Med. J.*, **307**, 1385–8

32. Wolfe, B.M. and Huff, M.W. (1993). Effect of low dosage progestin-only administration upon plasma triglycerides and lipoprotein metabolism in postmenopausal women. *J. Clin. Invest.*, **92**, 456–61

33. Stevenson, J.C. (1995). The metabolic and cardiovascular consequences of HRT. *Br. J. Clin. Pract.*, **49**, 87–90

34. Farrish, E., Rolton, H.A., Barnes, J.F. and Hart, D.M. (1991). Lipoprotein (a) concentrations in postmenopausal women taking norethisterone. *Br. Med. J.*, **303**, 694

35. Rymer, J., Crook, D., Sidhu, M., Chapman, M. and Stevenson, J.C. (1993). Effects of tibolone on serum concentrations of lipoprotein (a) in postmenopausal women. *Acta Endocrinol.*, **128**, 259–62

36. Marsh, M.S., Crook, D., Whitcroft, S.I.J., Worthington, M., Whitehead, M.I. and Stevenson, J.C. (1994). Effect of continuous combined estrogen and desogestrel replacement therapy on serum lipids and lipoproteins. *Obstet. Gynecol.*, **83**, 19–23

37. Stevenson, J.C., Crook, D., Godsland, I.F., Collins, P. and Whitehead, M.I. (1994). Hormone replacement therapy and the cardiovascular system. Nonlipid effects. *Drugs*, **47** (Suppl. 2), 35–41

3

Coagulation, fibrinolysis and hormone replacement therapy

G.D.O. Lowe

INTRODUCTION

The blood coagulation system is important in ensuring haemostasis when blood vessel integrity is challenged. On the other hand, excessive intravascular fibrin formation may result in thrombosis – arterial, venous or microcirculatory. Hence appropriate counterbalance to the coagulation system is normally provided not only by coagulation inhibitors (antithrombin and the protein C/protein S system) which prevent excessive fibrin formation, but also by the fibrinolytic system which prevents excessive fibrin accumulation. The key components of the coagulation and fibrinolytic systems are summarised in Figure 1.

In epidemiological studies, women have lower risks of both arterial and venous thromboembolism during their reproductive years and up to the age of 60 years, compared to men[1]. Possible reasons include the cardioprotective effects of physiological oestrogens, especially increased levels of high-density lipoprotein (HDL) cholesterol which may decrease atherogenesis[1]; decreased susceptibility to the effects of blood viscosity and fibrinogen on atherogenesis[2]; and lower haematocrit, which outweighs the effect of higher fibrinogen levels on blood viscosity[3]. However, after the age of 60 years, ischaemic heart disease (IHD) is the commonest cause of death in women: one in four women, as well as one in four men, die from

COAGULATION   FIBRINOLYSIS

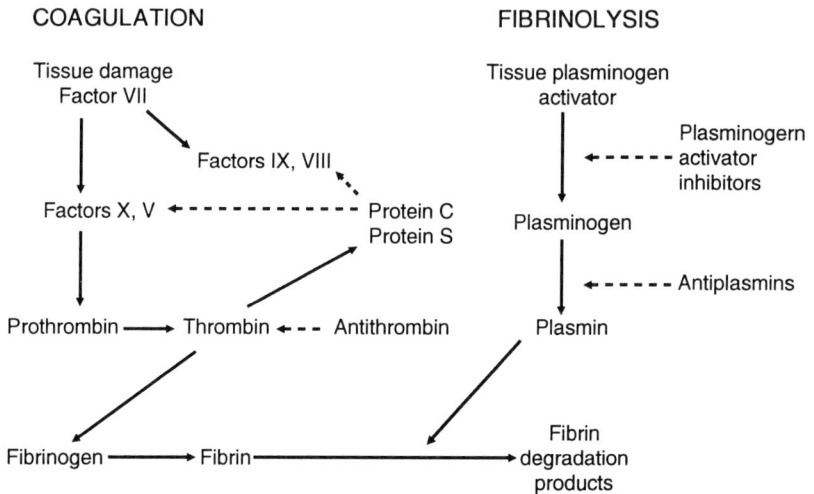

Figure 1 Key components of the blood coagulation and fibrinolytic systems

IHD (Figure 2)[1]. The narrowing gap between men and women in IHD risk (Figure 2) reflects not only increasing risk in post-menopausal women, but decelerated increase in risk in men, as well as earlier mortality in men[1]. Nevertheless, women with early sudden menopause (bilateral oophorectomy) who did not receive hormone replacement therapy (HRT) have a two-fold relative risk of IHD[4]. Furthermore, there is now compelling evidence that HRT reduces the risk of cardiovascular disease in post-menopausal women[1]. While this protective effect may be mediated partly through lipid metabolism, blood pressure, or insulin resistance, evidence from both cross-sectional studies[5–7] and from recently-reported prospective studies[8,10] indicates that reduction in plasma fibrinogen may be an important mechanism. HRT also has significant effects on levels of other coagulation factors, as well as on fibrinolytic factors[9,11]. There is increasing evidence that such factors are important predictors of both arterial and venous thrombosis[12].

The present review therefore aims to address the following questions:

(1)   Which coagulation or fibrinolysis variables are associated with increased cardiovascular risk?

30

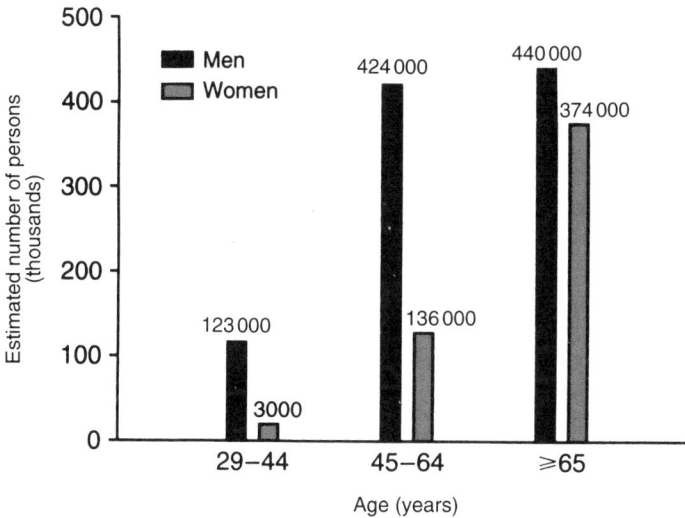

Figure 2 Annual incidence of myocardial infarction in women and men in the United States. From reference 1, with permission. Data from the Framingham Heart Study, adapted from the American Heart Association, Heart and Stroke Facts Statistics, 1992, with permission

(2)   What are the hormonal effects (gender, pregnancy, oral contraceptives, menopause, HRT) on these variables?

(3)   Are there any practical implications?

FIBRINOGEN

There is now much evidence that plasma fibrinogen is a strong and consistent predictor of cardiovascular events: ischaemic heart disease (IHD), stroke, peripheral arterial disease, venous thrombosis, atrial fibrillation and heart failure[13,14]. A meta-analysis of seven prospective studies of IHD and stroke found that persons in the highest third of plasma fibrinogen had a relative risk of 2.5 (95% confidence intervals, 2.0–2.8) compared to persons in the lowest third[15]. In the Scottish Heart Health Study[16], which has reported the largest number

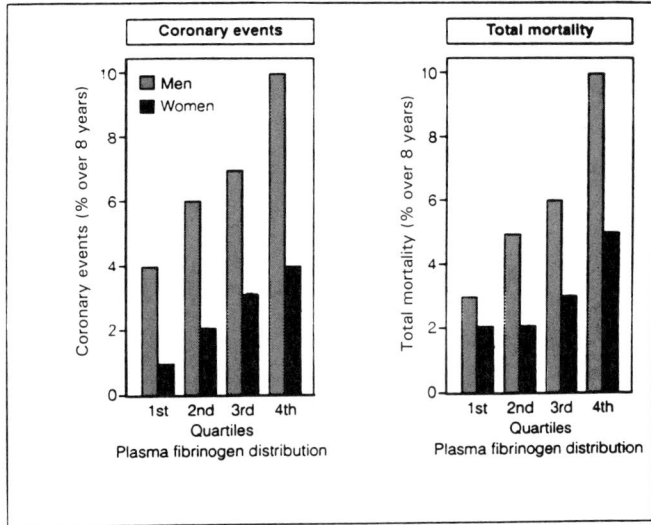

Figure 3 Increases in (left) ischaemic heart disease events; and (right) total mortality; with increasing plasma fibrinogen level in both men and women in the Scottish Heart Health Study. From reference 16, with permission

of events of any prospective study, fibrinogen was a strong predictor of both IHD events and total mortality in both men and women (Figure 3). Figure 3 shows that women aged 40–59 years in the highest quartile of plasma fibrinogen had a 4% risk of coronary events and a 5% risk of death over an average follow-up period of 8 years. Fibrinogen levels therefore merit evaluation in prediction of cardiovascular risk, together with other established risk predictors[14]. Fibrinogen is also a secondary predictor of cardiovascular events in persons with clinically established arterial disease[14].

Plasma fibrinogen is not only a risk predictor of cardiovascular events and death, but also a plausible mechanism through which certain risk factors (e.g. age, cigarette-smoking, diabetes, insulin resistance) and risk protectors (e.g. exercise, moderate alcohol consumption) may promote vascular disease. Fibrinogen infiltrates the arterial wall; promotes platelet aggregation and formation of platelet-fibrin thrombi; decreases the deformability and lysability of fibrin thrombi; and increases plasma and blood viscosity which may promote ischaemia. Stopping smoking, exercise, and control of diabetes can lower fibrinogen levels. Two large studies of secondary prevention with bezafibrate, which lowers plasma fibrinogen by about 25% as well as lowering cholesterol and triglyceride, are currently testing the hypothesis that fibrinogen reduction lowers the risk of cardiovascular events and death[14].

While women have slightly higher fibrinogen levels than men at all ages[6,14], the gradient of increasing risk of cardiovascular events with increasing fibrinogen in women appears lower than that in men (Figure 3). This may reflect a lower susceptibility to the effects of blood viscosity and fibrinogen on atherogenesis[2], or lower susceptibility to fibrinogen-mediated platelet aggregation[18]. Nevertheless, epidemiological studies suggest that lowering of plasma fibrinogen may be beneficial in cardiovascular risk-reduction in women as well as men (Figure 3).

Higher fibrinogen levels in women than men may be an oestrogenic effect, since fibrinogen levels are further elevated by combined oral contraceptives (Table 1) but not by progestin only preparations[6,20,21,22,27]. Fibrinogen levels also rise in pregnancy, especially in the last trimester; a further rise is seen in pregnancy-induced hypertension[23].

Fibrinogen levels rise after the menopause: however, in cross-sectional studies, users of hormone-replacement therapy had lower levels than non-users[5,6,7,25,26,28]. The prospective Postmenopausal Estrogen/Progestin Interventions (PEPI) Trial[8] as well as the Medical Research Council Trial[10] confirmed that HRT reduced the postmenopausal increase in fibrinogen, as well as decreasing low density lipoprotein (LDL) and increasing high density lipoprotein (HDL) cholesterol levels. In view of the predictive value of fibrinogen for cardiovascular events and mortality in women (Figure 3), this effect of HRT (which was observed in both unopposed oestrogen and combined oestrogen–progestin groups) may be one plausible mechanism for the apparent protective effects of HRT against cardiovascular disease.

Table 1 Mean age-adjusted fibrinogen and factor VII levels in women, according to use of combined oral contraceptives. Data from reference 25

	Oestrogen dose		
	None (*n* = 243)	30 µg (*n* = 15)	50 µg (*n* = 63)
Fibrinogen (g/l)	2.52	2.84	2.89
Factor VII (%)	83.0	96.6	121.1

FACTOR VII

Two prospective studies have shown that coagulation factor VII activity is a predictor of IHD events (especially fatal events) in men[27,29]. Whether or not factor VII is a risk predictor for IHD in women is not yet known. There is no evidence that factor VII is a risk factor for venous thromboembolism[13]. Factor VII is related to dietary fat intake, obesity, dyslipidaemia and glucose intolerance; hence it is one potential link between these risk predictors and arterial thrombosis[30]. Ongoing studies of low-dose warfarin (which lowers factor VII activity) in high-risk men are testing the causality of this association[30].

As with fibrinogen, factor VII activity levels are higher in combined oral contraceptive users, but not in progestin-only users: the effects of oestrogen appear dose-dependent above 30 µg/day[19,25] (Table 1). Factor VII levels also increase in pregnancy[31].

Factor VII activity increases after the menopause[25]. In a large cross-sectional study, users of unopposed oestrogen HRT had higher levels of factor VII than non-users or oestrogen-progestin users, possibly associated with higher triglyceride levels[7] (Table 2). This finding is in keeping with several small prospective studies[9,32] and one large study[10] (Figure 4). In one study, the combination of 2 mg 17β-oestradiol and 1 mg norethisterone acetate was found to *lower* factor VII activity and antigen[33]. It therefore appears that progestins may prevent or reverse the tendency of oestrogen replacement therapy to increase factor VII activity levels; possibly through their effects on lipid metabolism. This possibility is supported by the results

Table 2 Cross-sectional associations of coagulation factors (adjusted means) and HRT in postmenopausal women. Data from reference 7. NS = not statistically significant

	HRT users		*HRT non-users*		*p values*	
	Group (1) *Oestrogen*	*Group (2)* *Combined*	*Group (3)* *Ex-users*	*Group (4)* *Never*	*(1) vs. (2)*	*(1) + (2) vs. (3) + (4)*
Fibrinogen (g/l)	2.98	2.98	3.10	3.15	NS	0.001
Factor VII (%)	136	127	126	125	0.001	0.001
Triglyceride (mg/dl)	141	131	123	120	0.1	0.001
Factor VIII (%)	134	132	133	136	NS	NS
Von Willebrand factor (%)	119	118	119	121	NS	NS
Antithrombin (%)	110	113	114	115	0.17	0.002
Protein C (μg/ml)	3.47	3.30	3.29	3.27	0.001	0.001

of the Medical Research Council Study[10] (Figure 4). The increase in factor VII activity induced by mestranol was maintained for 20 years in one study[9].

FACTOR VIII/VON WILLEBRAND FACTOR

As with factor VII, recent studies suggest that factor VIII activity, which is closely correlated with plasma levels of its carrier protein von Willebrand factor (VWF), is a predictor of both IHD[34,35] and venous thrombosis[36]. A causal role for factor VIII in thrombosis is suggested by the low risk of thrombosis in haemophilia A[37]. Von Willebrand factor may promote thrombosis not only by increasing plasma factor VIII levels, but also by promoting platelet adhesion and aggregation.

As with fibrinogen and factor VII, plasma levels of factor VIII and von Willebrand factor may rise in users of combined oral contraceptives; and also in pregnancy[31]. These effects are beneficial in reduc-

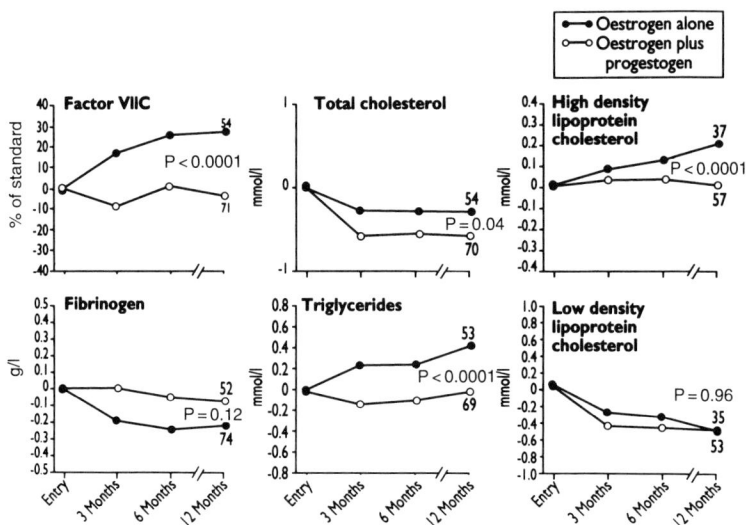

Figure 4 Changes in plasma fibrinogen, factor VII, and lipids/lipoproteins in a randomized trial of unopposed oestrogen and combined oestrogen-progestin hormone replacement therapy (HRT). From reference 10, with permission. Compare the effects of HRT on fibrinogen and factor VII with those of COCs (Table 1)

ing the risk of excessive bleeding in many women who have von Willebrand's disease or who are symptomatic carriers of haemophilia A[38].

Factor VIII and VWF also increase after the menopause; however, neither unopposed-oestrogen nor oestrogen-progestin HRT appear to have any effect[7] (Table 2).

COAGULATION INHIBITORS

Deficiencies of antithrombin, protein C or protein S are associated with venous thromboembolism, which may be precipitated by pregnancy or combined oral contraceptives[39,40]. Their associations with arterial disease are not well-established[24,39]. Antithrombin levels are higher in postmenopausal women than men[24], while protein S levels are lower in women than men at all ages[41]. Combined oral contraceptives tend to reduce antithrombin levels[19,25] and protein S levels[41], but to increase protein C levels[19]. In pregnancy, protein S levels fall, while antithrombin and protein C levels show no overall change[31].

Unopposed oestrogen HRT appears to reduce antithrombin levels and increase protein C levels; while oestrogen-progestin HRT appears to have no effect[7] (Table 2). However, no effect of mestranol on antithrombin levels was seen after 20 years[42].

Recently there has been great interest in activated protein C (APC) resistance: a reduction in the ability of APC to shorten the activated partial thromboplastin time (APTT) which often reflects a mutation in coagulation factor V (V Leiden: *Arg* 506 *Glu*) which reduces its inactivation by APC[43,44]. The presence of this congenital thrombophilia increases the risk of venous (but not arterial) thrombosis[45,46]. Vandenbroucke and colleagues[47] recently observed that factor V Leiden is associated with increased risk of venous thromboembolism during contraceptive pill usage.

FIBRINOLYSIS

Women have higher fibrinolytic potential of the blood than men, and a further increase if they use oral contraceptive pills[25]. This reflects lower levels of the fibrinolytic inhibitor, plasminogen activator inhibitor type 1 (PAI-1) which complexes with and inhibits tissue-type plasminogen activator (tPA); as a result, women have lower levels of plasma tPA antigen, much of which circulates as inactive tPA–PAI-1 complexes[27,48]. Plasminogen levels also increase with oestrogen use. In pregnancy, plasminogen increases and fibrinolytic potential falls, due not only to increase in PAI-1, but also to a marked increase in placentally-derived plasminogen activator inhibitor type 2 (PAI-2)[31].

Fibrinolytic potential decreases after the menopause, due to increase in PAI-1[48]. HRT increases fibrinolytic potential by reducing PAI-1 (and hence tPA antigen) levels[9,27,32,49]. As with factor VII, this effect was maintained for 20 years in one study of mestranol[9].

MARKERS OF ACTIVATED COAGULATION AND FIBRINOLYSIS

Recent studies have suggested that users of combined oral contraceptive pills have increased plasma levels of activation markers of both coagulation (e.g. fibrinopeptide A, prothrombin fragment F1 + 2, thrombin-antithrombin complexes) and fibrinolysis (e.g. fibrin(ogen) degradation products[27,49]. Similar changes are observed in pregnancy, as well as during HRT with oestrogen[49,50]. These findings suggest that oestrogens activate both blood coagulation and fibrinolysis, possibly achieving a "balance" at a higher equilibrium.

PRACTICAL IMPLICATIONS

(1)   Gender differences in both blood coagulation and fibrinolysis may be relevant to the lower risk of cardiovascular events in women than men; and in the increase in risk after the menopause. Overall, the effects of HRT on coagulation (as well as metabolism) suggest a favourable effect on cardiovascular risk[7,10]; and the profibrinolytic effect of HRT may also be favourable. These effects of HRT are modified by progestins[7,10]. Whether or not these effects are translated into cardiovascular protection (as suggested by observational studies) will only be established by the large randomized trials of unopposed oestrogen and oestrogen-progestin HRT which are currently in progress[10]. Both coagulation and fibrinolysis should be studied in such trials.

(2)   Pregnancy has marked effects on both blood coagulation and fibrinolysis, which may be relevant to the increased risk of venous thromboembolism in pregnancy and the puerperium. Guidelines for the identification of women at increased risk, and for antithrombotic prophylaxis, have recently been published[51,52].

REFERENCES

1. Rich-Edwards, J.W., Manson, J.E., Hennekens, C.H. and Buring, J.E. (1995). The primary prevention of coronary heart disease in women. *N. Engl. J. Med.*, **332**, 1758–66
2. Fowkes, F.G.R., Pell, J.P., Donnan, P.T. *et al.* (1994). Sex differences in susceptibility to etiologic factors for peripheral atherosclerosis – importance of blood viscosity and plasma fibrinogen. *Arterioscler. Thromb.*, **14**, 862–5
3. Lowe, G.D.O. (1994). Blood rheology and vascular disease. In Bloom, A.L., Forbes, C.D., Thomas, D.P. and Tuddenham, E.G.D. (eds.) *Haemostasis and Thrombosis*, 3rd edn., pp. 1169–88. (Edinburgh: Churchill Livingstone)
4. Colditz, C.A., Willett, W.C., Stampfer, M.J., Rosner, B., Speizer, F.E., Hennekens, C.H. (1987). Menopause and the risk of coronary heart disease in women. *N. Engl. J. Med.*, **316**, 1105–10
5. Meilahn, E.N., Kuller, L.H., Matthews, K.A., Kiss, J.E. (1992). Variation in plasma fibrinogen levels by menopausal status and use of hormone replacement therapy: the Healthy Women Study. In Ernst, E., Koenig, W., Lowe, G.D.O., Meade, T.W. (eds.) *Fibrinogen: a "new" cardiovascular risk factor*, pp. 338–43. (Vienna: Blackwell MZV)
6. Lee, A.J., Lowe, G.D.O., Smith, W.C.S. and Tunstall-Pedoe, H. (1993). Plasma fibrinogen in women: relationships with oral contraceptives, the menopause and hormone replacement therapy. *Br. J. Haematol.*, **83**, 616–21
7. Nabulsi, A.A., Folsom, A.R., White, A. *et al.* (1993). Association of hormone replacement therapy with various cardiovascular risk factors in postmenopausal women. *N. Engl. J. Med.*, **328**, 1069–75
8. PEPI Trial (1995). Effects of estrogen or estrogen/progestin regimes on heart disease risk factors in postmenopausal women: the Postmenopausal Estrogen/Progestin Interventions (PEPI) Trial. *J. Am. Med. Assoc.*, **273**, 199–208
9. Lowe, G.D.O., Spowart, K.J.M. and Rumley, A. (1993). Epidemiological and clinical studies of hemostasis, the menopause and hormone replacement therapy. *Gynecol. Endocrinol.*, **7**, Suppl., 71–4
10. Medical Research Council, General Practice Research Framework (1996). Randomised comparison of oestrogen *versus* oestrogen plus progestogen hormone replacement therapy in women with hysterectomy. *Br. Med. J.*, **312**, 473–8
11. Stevenson, J.C., Crook, D., Godsland, I.F., Collins, P. and Whitehead, M.I. (1994). Hormone replacement therapy and the cardiovascular system. Non lipid effects. *Drugs*, **47**, Suppl., 35–41

12. Lowe, G.D.O. (1996). Haemostatic risk factors for arterial and venous thrombosis. In Poller, L. and Ludlam, C.A. (eds.) *Recent Advances in Blood Coagulation*, 7, pp. 67–94. (Edinburgh: Churchill Livingstone)

13. Koster, T., Rosendaal, F.R., Reitsma, P.H., van der Velden, P.A., Briët, E. and Vandenbroucke, J.P. (1994). Factor VII and fibrinogen levels as risk factors for venous thrombosis. A case–control study of plasma levels and DNA polymorphisms. Leiden Thrombophilia Study (LETS). *Thromb. Haemostas.*, **71**, 719–22

14. Lowe, G.D.O., Fowkes, F.G.R., Koenig, W. and Mannucci, P.M. (eds.) (1995). Fibrinogen and cardiovascular disease. *Eur. Heart J.*, **16**, Supplement A

15. Resch, K.L. and Ernst, E. (1995). The complex impact of fibrinogen on atherosclerosis-related diseases. In Koenig, W., Hornbach, V., Bond, M.G. and Kramsch, D.M. (eds.). *Progression and Regression of Atherosclerosis*, pp. 36–40. (Vienna: Blackwell MZV)

16. Lowe, G.D.O. (1996). Risk factors in cardiovascular disease. In Cleland, J. (ed.) *Asymptomatic Coronary Artery Disease and Angina*, pp. 13–27. (London: Science Press)

17. Lee, A.J., Smith, W.C.S., Lowe, G.D.O. *et al.* (1990). Plasma fibrinogen and coronary risk factors: the Scottish Heart Health Study. *J. Clin. Epidemiol.*, **43**, 913–19

18. Meade, T.W., Vickers, M.V., Thompson, S.G. *et al.* (1985). Epidemiological characteristics of platelet aggregability. *Br. Med. J.*, **290**, 428–32

19. Heinrich, J., Schulte, H. and Asmann, G. (1993). Oral contraceptives and variables of coagulation and fibrinolysis in an epidemiological study. *Gynecol. Endocrinol.*, **7**, Suppl. 55–8

20. Meade, T.W., Chakrabarti, R., Haines, A.P., North, W.R.S. and Stirling, Y. (1979). Characteristics affecting fibrinolytic activity and plasma fibrinogen concentration. *Br. Med. J.*, **1**, 153–6

21. Balleisen, L., Bailey, J., Epping, P.H., Schulte, H. and van de Loo, J. (1985). Epidemiological study on factor VII, factor VIII and fibrinogen in an industrial population. I. Baseline data on the relation to age, gender, body-weight, smoking, alcohol, pill-using, and menopause. *Thromb. Haemostas.*, **54**, 475–9

22. Folsom, A.R., Qambiek, H.T., Flack, J.M. *et al.* for the investigators of the Coronary Artery Risk Development in Young Adults (CARDIA) Study (1993). Plasma fibrinogen: levels and correlates in young adults. *Am. J. Epidemiol.*, **138**, 1023–36

23. Lowe, G.D.O. (1992). Blood rheology in pregnancy – physiology and pathology. In Greer, I.A., Turpie, A.G.G. and Forbes, C.D. (eds.)

Haemostasis and Thrombosis in Obstetrics and Gynaecology, pp. 27–44. (London: Chapman and Hall)

24. Meade, T.W., Dyer, S., Howarth, D.J., Imeson, J.D. and Stirling, Y. (1991). Antithrombin III and procoagulant activity: sex differences and effects of the menopause. *Br. J. Haematol.*, **74**, 77–81

25. Meade, T.W. (1990). Oestrogens and thrombosis. In Drife, J.O. and Studd, J.W.W. (eds.) *Hormone Replacement Therapy and Osteoporosis*, pp. 223–33. (Berlin: Springer Verlag)

26. Folsom, A.R., Wu, K.K., Davis, C.E., Conlan, M.G., Sorlie, P.D. and Szklo, M. (1991). Population correlates of plasma fibrinogen and factor VII, putative cardiovascular risk factors. *Atherosclerosis*, **91**, 191–205

27. Henrich, J., Balleisen, L., Schulte, H. *et al.* (1994). Fibrinogen and factor VII in the prediction of coronary risk. Results from the PROCAM study in healthy men. *Arterioscler. Thromb.*, **14**, 54–9

28. Scarabin, P.Y., Plu-Bureau, G., Bara, L., Bonithon-Kopp, C., Guize, L. and Samama, M.M. (1993). Haemostatic variables and menopausal status: influence of hormone replacement therapy. *Thromb. Haemostas.*, **70**, 584–5

29. Ruddock, V. and Meade, T.W. (1994). Factor VII activity and ischaemic heart disease: fatal and non-fatal events. *Q. J. Med.*, **87**, 403–6

30. Meade, T.W. (1995). *Haemostatic Variables, Thrombosis and Ischaemic Heart Disease*. (Amsterdam: Excerpta Medica)

31. Forbes, C.D. and Greer, I.A. (1992). Physiology of haemostasis and the effect of pregnancy. In Greer, I.A., Turpie, A.G.G., Forbes, C.D. (eds.). *Haemostasis and Thrombosis in Obstetrics and Gynaecology*, pp. 1–25. (London: Chapman and Hall)

32. Stanwell-Smith, R. and Meade, T.W. (1984). Hormone replacement therapy for menopausal women: a review of its effects on haemostatic function, lipids, and blood pressure. *Adv. Drug React. Ac. Pois. Rev.*, **4**, 187–210

33. Sporrong, T., Mattsson, L-A., Samsoe, G., Stigendal, L. and Hellgren, M. (1990). Haemostatic changes during continuous oestradiol-progestogen treatment of postmenopausal women. *Br. J. Obstet. Gynaecol.*, **97**, 939–44

34. Meade, T.W., Cooper, J.C., Stirling, Y. *et al.* (1994). Factor VIII, ABO blood group and the incidence of ischaemic heart disease. *Br. J. Haematol.*, **88**, 601–7

35. Lowe, G.D.O., Rumley, A., Yarnell, J.W.G. and Sweetnam, P.M. (1995). Fibrin D-dimer, von Willebrand factor, tissue plasminogen activator antigen, and plasminogen activator inhibitor activity are primary risk factors for ischaemic heart disease: the Caerphilly Study. *Thromb. Haemostas.*, **73**, 950

36. Koster, T., Blann, A.D., Briët, E., Vandenbroucke, J.P. and Rosendaal, F.R. (1995). Role of clotting factor VIII in effect of von Willebrand factor on occurrence of deep vein thrombosis. *Lancet*, **345**, 152–5
37. Rosendaal, F.R., Varekamp, I., Smit, C. *et al.* (1989). Mortality and causes of death in Dutch haemophiliacs, 1973–86. *Br. J. Haematol.*, **71**, 71–6
38. Greer, I.A., Lowe, G.D.O., Walker, J.J. and Forbes, C.D. (1991). Haemorrhagic problems in obstetrics and gynaecology in patients with congenital coagulopathies. *Br. J. Obstet. Gynaecol.*, **98**, 909–18
39. Allaart, C.F. and Briët, E. (1994). Familial venous thrombophilia. In Bloom, A.L., Forbes, C.D., Thomas, D.P. and Tuddenham, E.G.D. (eds.) *Haemostasis and Thrombosis*, 3rd edn., pp. 1349–60. (Edinburgh: Churchill Livingstone)
40. Koster, T. (1995). *Deep-vein thrombosis. A population-based case-control study: Leiden Thrombophilia Study.* Thesis, University of Leiden, The Netherlands
41. Boerger, L.M., Morris, P.C., Thurnase, G.R., Esmon, C.T. and Comp, P.C. (1987). Oral contraceptives and gender affect protein S status. *Blood*, **69**, 692–4
42. Al-Azzawi, F., Smith, D., Parkin, D., Hart, D.M. and Lindsay, R. (1989). Blood coagulation profile in long-term hormone replacement therapy with mestranol. *Maturitas*, **11**, 95–101
43. Bertina, R.M., Reitsma, P.H., Rosendaal, F.R. and Vandenbroucke, J.P. (1995). Resistance to activated protein C and factor V Leiden as risk factors for venous thrombosis. *Thromb. Haemostas.*, **74**, 449–53
44. Dahlback, B. (1995). New molecular insights into the genetics of thrombophilia. *Thromb. Haemostas.*, **74**, 139–48
45. Koster, T., Rosendaal, F.R., de Ronde, H., Briët, E., Vandenbroucke, J.P. and Bertina, R.M. (1993). Venous thrombosis due to poor anticoagulant response to activated protein C: Leiden Thrombophilia Study. *Lancet*, **362**, 1503–6
46. Ridker, P.M., Hennekens, C.H., Lindpaintner, K. *et al.* (1995). Mutation in the gene coding for coagulation factor V and the risk of myocardial infarction, stroke, and venous thrombosis in apparently healthy men. *N. Engl. J. Med.*, **332**, 912–7
47. Vandenbroucke, J.P., Koster, T., Briët, E., Reitsma, R.M., Bertina, R.M. and Rosendaal, F.R. (1994). Increased risk of venous thrombosis in oral-contraceptive users who are carriers of factor V Leiden mutation. *Lancet*, **344**, 1453–7
48. Eliasson, M. (1995). *The epidemiology of fibrinogen and fibrinolysis.* MD Thesis, University of Umeå, Sweden

49. Winkler, U.H. (1992). Menopause, hormone replacement therapy and cardiovascular disease: a review of haemostaseological findings. *Fibrinolysis*, **6**, Suppl. 3: 5–10
50. Bauer, K.A., Rosenberg, R.D. (1994). Activation makers of coagulation. *Baillière's Clin. Haematol.*, **7**, 523–40
51. British Society for Haematology. (1993). Guidelines on the prevention, investigation, and management of thrombosis associated with pregnancy. *J. Clin. Pathol.*, **46**, 489–96
52. Scottish Intercollegiate Guidelines Network (SIGN). (1995). Prophylaxis of Venous Thromboembolism. (Edinburgh: SIGN)

4

Bone mineral density measurements: advances and problems

I. Fogelman and G.M. Blake

INTRODUCTION

At the present time dual X-ray absorptiometry (DXA) is the most widely used technique for measuring bone mineral density (BMD). Compared with the earlier technique of dual photon absorptiometry (DPA), based on a Gd-153 radionuclide source, DXA has the advantages of high precision, short scanning times, low radiation dose and stable calibration in the clinical environment[1-3]. While the spine is the most frequently measured site, there are a wide variety of additional applications now available. These include BMD measurements of the proximal femur, distal forearm and total body together with specialist applications such as body composition and vertebral morphometry. As a result the past 5 years have seen the rapid expansion of both research and routine clinical studies based on DXA[4.]

The replacement of the Gd-153 radionuclide source with an X-ray tube improved the performance of dual photon absorptiometry by combining high photon flux with the small focal-spot size at the anode of the X-ray tube. The availability of an intense, narrow beam of radiation improved scanning time and image definition and led to a concomitant improvement in precision.

The first generation of DXA scanners used a pencil beam coupled to a single detector in the scanning arm. An important development in DXA technology was the introduction of scanners with a fan beam coupled to a linear array of detectors[5,6] (Figure 1). Fan-beam studies are acquired by the scanning arm performing a single sweep across the patient instead of the two-dimensional raster scan required by pencil-beam geometry. As a result, scan times have been significantly shortened. A number of studies have demonstrated the equivalence of pencil- and fan-beam BMD measurements[7,8].

A major motivation behind the recent developments is the desire for DXA scanners to be capable of producing vertebral-morphometry studies with high resolution and short scan times.

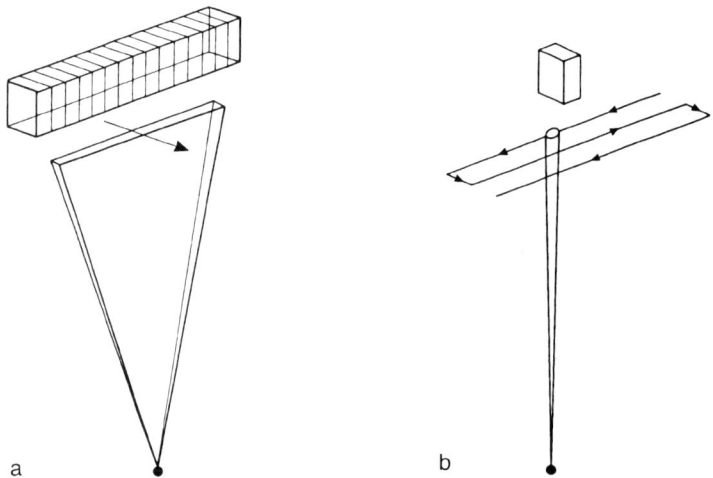

Figure 1 Comparison of X-ray beam and detector geometry for a fan-beam configuration with a multidetector array (a) and a pencil-beam configuration with a single detector (b)

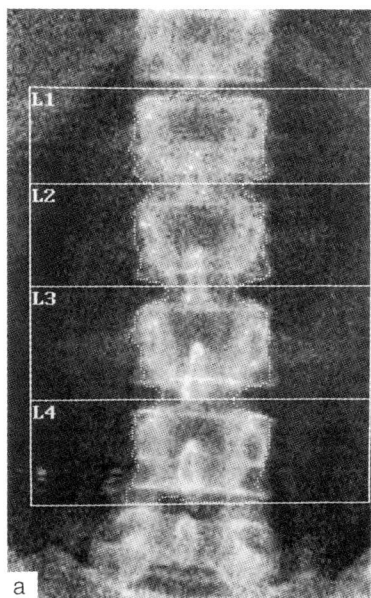

Region	Area (cm^2)	BMC (g)	BMD (g/cm^2)
L1	12.85	10.01	0.779
L2	13.90	11.38	0.819
L3	14.81	11.52	0.778
L4	14.88	12.71	0.854
Total	56.44	45.61	0.808

b

Figure 2 A posteroanterior (PA) projection DXA scan of the lumbar spine in a postmenopausal patient (a) with results of bone mineral content (BMC) and bone mineral density (BMD) measurements (b). Area BMD expressed in units of grams of hydroxyapatite per square centimetre of projected area is measured for the individual vertebrae L1 to L4 and is then averaged over their total area

DXA APPLICATIONS

Posteroanterior lumbar spine and hip

The scanning software developed for first-generation DXA systems provided for clinical studies using posteroanterior (PA) projection scans of the lumbar spine (Figure 2) and proximal femur. It is usual to examine BMD in the hip in three regions: the femoral neck, the greater trochanter and Ward's triangle (Figure 3). The latter measures the earliest site of postmenopausal bone loss in the proximal femur and is of interest because in principle it gives the best measure of trabecular bone in the hip. In practice, however, use of the Ward's triangle region is limited by the poor precision of measurements at this site and the femoral neck is the region usually used.

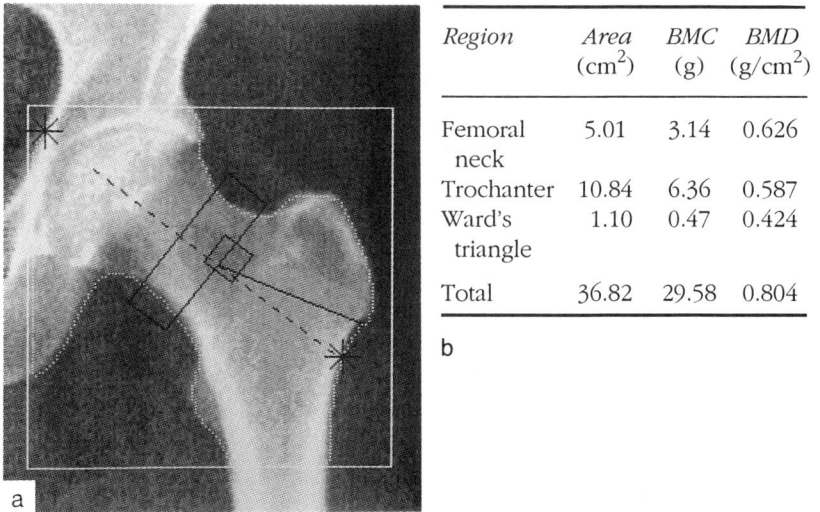

Region	Area (cm^2)	BMC (g)	BMD (g/cm^2)
Femoral neck	5.01	3.14	0.626
Trochanter	10.84	6.36	0.587
Ward's triangle	1.10	0.47	0.424
Total	36.82	29.58	0.804

Figure 3 A DXA scan of the proximal femur (a). The hip analysis software generates bone mineral content (BMC) and bone mineral density (BMD) measurements (b) in the femoral neck (oblong box), Ward's triangle (small square box) and the greater trochanter (above the solid diagonal line)

The spine can be measured with high precision but is subject to artefacts, particularly in the elderly, such as co-existent degenerative disease, which can artificially elevate values. This is much less of a problem in the femoral neck but measurements are technically more difficult and care must be taken that the patient is correctly positioned to avoid any rotation and also with the analysis, e.g. where the region of interest (ROI) is placed. Such factors lead to poorer precision for the femoral neck than the spine (typically 2% and 1%, respectively).

For the majority of clinical studies DXA scans of the PA spine and hip provide sufficient information. However, developments in DXA have made available new scanning modes and specialized applications that supplement the conventional spine and hip studies.

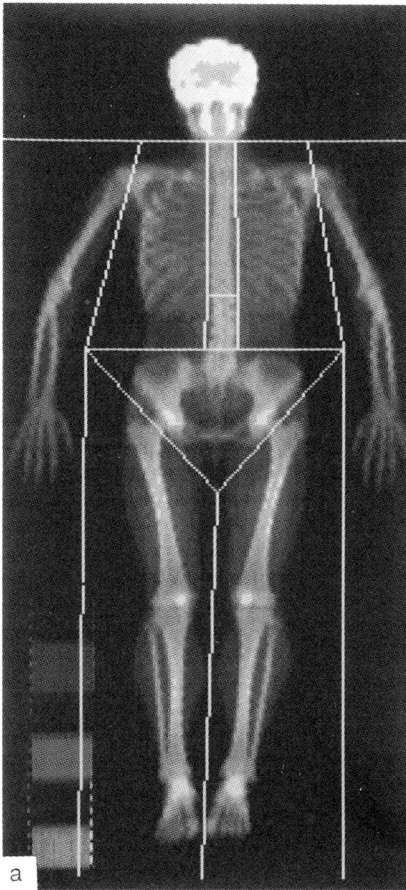

Region	Area (cm^2)	BMC (g)	BMD (g/cm^2)
Left arm	175.6	144.6	0.823
Right arm	189.7	150.4	0.793
Left ribs	148.6	104.0	0.700
Right ribs	138.1	95.0	0.688
Thoracic spine	141.4	142.8	1.010
Lumbar spine	50.3	61.1	1.213
Pelvis	231.6	286.5	1.237
Left leg	360.5	444.4	1.233
Right leg	367.3	459.1	1.250
Head	255.7	640.8	2.506
Total	2058.8	2528.6	1.228

b

a

Figure 4 A DXA scan of the total skeleton (a). As well as measuring bone mineral content (BMC) and bone mineral density (BMD) over the whole body, results are given separately for 10 subregions in the skeleton (b). From the same scan the body composition software will also estimate total body and subregional fat and lean-tissue masses

Distal forearm

Studies of the radius are performed by placing the non-dominant forearm on the scanning table and scanning the distal half from the midradius to the wrist. Unlike single photon absorptiometry (SPA) or single X-ray absorptiometry (SXA) studies, DXA scans of the forearm can be performed in air and do not require the use of a water bath.

Total body studies

Total body DXA is of interest because of the comprehensive view it affords of changes across the whole skeleton (Figure 4). Whole-body scans measure bone mineral content (BMC) and average BMD in the total skeleton together with subregions that include the skull, arms, ribs, thoracic and lumbar spine, pelvis and legs[9].

An interesting new application made possible by total-body DXA is body-composition studies[9,10]. In those areas of a whole-body scan where the X-ray beam does not intersect bone it is possible to use the attenuation of the two photon energies to measure separately the masses of fat and lean tissue. Over bone, however, only BMD and total (fat and lean) soft-tissue mass can be measured. Extrapolation of measurements of the percentage of body fat in soft tissue over adjacent bone means that a whole-body DXA scan can provide estimates of total-body fat and lean mass as well as BMD.

Prosthetic implants

Another specialized application under evaluation is the study of the integrity of hip prostheses. In such patients scanning of the hip is complicated by the high X-ray attenuation of the metal implant. Software can now identify and reject the prosthesis and automatically place ROIs around the periprosthetic bone[11]. Studies are underway to determine whether serial-DXA scanning after hip replacement can identify mechanical loosening and the durability of implants[12] and so aid improvements in the design of future implants.

Lateral lumbar spine

The rapid turnover of the metabolically-active trabecular bone in the vertebral bodies makes the spine the optimum site for monitoring changes in bone mineralization[13]. DXA scans of the lumbar spine using the lateral instead of the PA projection isolate the vertebral bodies from the posterior elements and better approximate the objective of measuring trabecular bone free of artefacts.

Initial lateral DXA studies were performed using the decubitus method in which subjects lie on their side[14,15]. While first reports gave precisions with a coefficient of variation (CV) of 2–3%, later studies gave 5–6%[16]. The poor precision of the decubitus scan is partly the result of the difficulty in reproducing subjects' positions on follow-up scans which leads to variation in the thickness and composition of the soft-tissue baseline. An important development in lateral studies has been the introduction of the new generation of fan-beam systems equipped with a rotating scanning arm. This enables the lateral scan to be performed with the patient in supine position.

Use of the supine position and baseline-compensation algorithm has improved the short-term precision of vertebral-body BMD measurements to 1%[6,16] and the technique may have a use in clinical trials.

Vertebral morphometry

Recent prospective clinical trials of new treatments for osteoporosis have given increased emphasis to the primary objective of such studies of demonstrating that therapies are successful in reducing the incidence of fragility fractures. Spinal crush fractures are an important sequelae of osteoporosis and it is usual to monitor the incidence of new vertebral deformities by performing serial morphometric measurements of vertebral-body height on lateral radiographs of the lumbar and thoracic spine[17–19].

The latest fan-beam DXA systems are designed to perform fast high-resolution lateral scans of the lumbar and thoracic spine (L4–T4) acquired with the patient in the supine position (Figure 5). A major advantage of DXA systems for vertebral morphometry is the elimination of the geometrical distortion associated with lateral radiographs that arises from the X-ray cone beam and can cause errors due to variable projection and magnification[20]. A further significant advantage is the much lower radiation dose to the patient

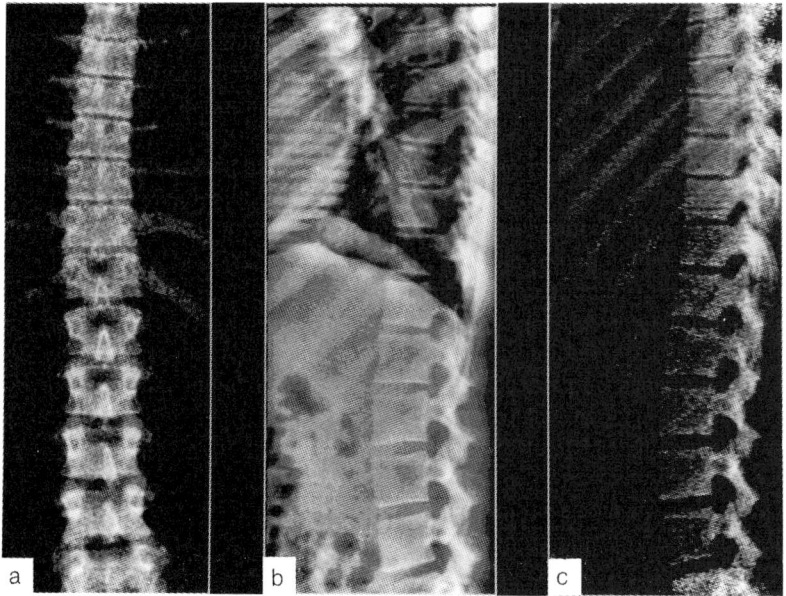

Figure 5 High resolution lateral scans of the lumbar and thoracic spine (L4–T4) can be used for morphometric X-ray absorptiometry (MXA) studies of vertebral deformities. These images were produced on a Hologic QDR-4500 system. An initial PA scan of the spine (a) generates a centreline in the middle of the spine which is tracked during the lateral scan to eliminate magnification errors. Both dual-energy (c) and single-energy (b) lateral images are available for analysis

from DXA compared with radiographs. Initial studies of DXA vertebral morphometry have shown good agreement with radiographic studies after allowing for the elimination of the magnification error. If DXA can be shown to give adequate image quality for reliably identifying vertebral deformities morphometry would be a major rationale for its use in future clinical trials and for monitoring patients with established spinal osteoporosis.

PRECISION

Precision errors are defined to characterize the reproducibility of a diagnostic technique. Accuracy errors, on the other hand, reflect the degree to which measured results deviate from true values. Despite the obvious importance of validating the accuracy of bone-densitometry techniques, only a few studies of DPA or DXA have addressed this issue[21–24]. However, despite the general lack of accuracy data, for studies of patients receiving treatment for osteoporosis, it is usually precision that is the more important factor since it is essential to be able to reliably measure changes after a short-time interval.

Short-term precision

Most studies of equipment or new techniques include a measurement of short-term precision[6,9,14,16,25,26]. This involves performing a number of repeated measurements on a representative set of individuals to characterize the reproducibility of the technique. Generally, short-term precision errors are assessed from measurements performed either on the same day or extending over a period of no more than 2 weeks. Since true changes in BMD may confound measurements made over a longer period of time, the assessment of short-term and long-term precision require different treatment of the data.

Short-term precision is evaluated by taking the mean and variance of two or more repeated measurements on each subject. The individual means and variances for all the subjects are then averaged and the root mean square standard deviation (RMS SD) calculated[16]. For many purposes the absolute error expressed by the RMS SD is the most satisfactory definition of short-term precision. However, it is a popular convention to express precision data as the coefficient of variation (CV) by dividing the standard deviation by the mean for all subjects and expressing the result as a percentage:

$$CV = \frac{RMS\ SD\ (x)}{x} \times 100\%$$

The reason why many authors prefer to use CV rather than SD to express precision data is probably because the significance of a result given as a CV is more readily comprehended.

Long-term precision

The assessment of the long-term reproducibility of a technique is complicated by the fact that the variations in the data will reflect true changes in bone mineral as well as imprecision in the measurements. Use of the standard deviation to express the long-term precision would therefore result in an overestimate of the true precision errors of the technique.

In many subjects the plot of bone density against time approximates closely to a linear change. A parameter that quantifies the sources of variability over and above the true linear change is the standard error of the estimate (SEE) obtained from linear regression analysis of the data. However, the SEE will still include any variability due to non-linear changes in bone density and therefore may not be appropriate in subjects who have recently commenced or discontinued treatment for osteoporosis. As with short-term precision, results from different individuals are combined to find the RMS average SEE. In a manner analogous to short-term precision, the long-term precision may be expressed as the coefficient of variation by dividing the RMS SEE by the mean for all subjects and expressing the result as a percentage:

$$CV = \frac{RMS\ SEE\ (x)}{x} \times 100\%$$

Long-term precision is a more realistic parameter for assessing the significance of changes measured in longitudinal studies than short-term precision. Even when the underlying changes in bone mineral are truly linear, long-term precision would be expected to exceed short-term precision due to small drifts in instrumental calibration, variations in patient positioning and changes in soft-tissue composition. Typically, in many studies long-term precision is around twice the short-term precision.

CLINICAL STUDIES OF BONE DENSITY

What is normal?

One of the difficulties of interpreting the results of bone densitometry is that there is little consensus on how BMD measurements should be presented. To be clinically useful, BMD results for individual patients must be related to similar values obtained from a healthy

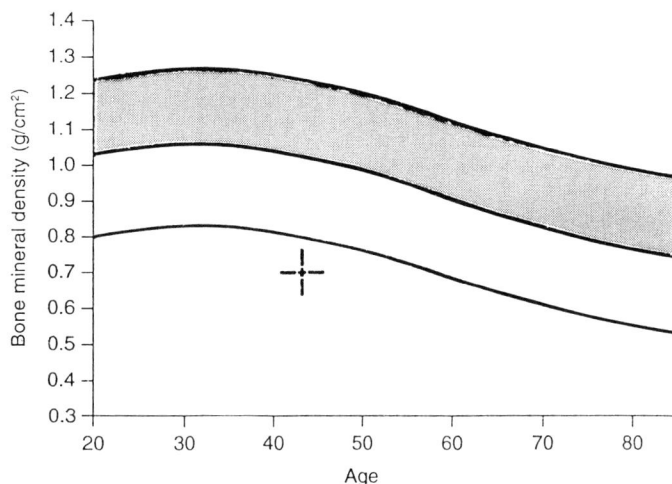

Figure 6 Posteroanterior lumbar spine bone mineral density (BMD) for a perimenopausal patient plotted with the normal reference curves. The middle curve shows the mean BMD in normal subjects ($Z = 0$) while the upper and lower curves show the ± 2 standard deviation limits ($Z = \pm 2$). This patient was recommended to commence oestrogen replacement therapy

reference population. The reference population is usually described in terms of the mean BMD and the population standard deviation (SD) matched for age, sex and race. A convenient method of displaying the results for an individual patient is to use a diagram in which the reference population is shown as the mean ± 2 SD (Figure 6). Provided the reference data are accurate and appropriate, 95% of normal subjects will lie within the ± 2 SD limits. The advantage of the plot shown in Figure 6 is that the interpretation of the measured BMD relative to the reference range is immediately apparent.

The Z-score

The information given visually in Figure 6 can also be expressed numerically by using Z-scores. The Z-score is defined by the equation:

$$Z\text{-score} = \frac{\text{Measured BMD} - \text{Age matched mean BMD}}{\text{Population standard deviation}}$$

and expresses by how many standard deviations a subject differs from the mean value for an age, sex and race matched reference population. Thus a subject lying on the central curve in Figure 6 has a Z-score or zero, while subjects on the upper and lower curves have Z-scores of +2 and –2, respectively. An advantage of the Z-score is that although different manufacturer's instruments may have different normal ranges for BMD due to differences in technology, edge-detection algorithms and calibration, Z-score results should be identical provided that comparable reference populations are used.

A potential limitation of using Z-scores derived from age-dependent reference data like that shown in Figure 6 is that the smooth variation of mean BMD and SD with age makes no allowance for whether a subject is pre-, peri- or postmenopausal or the number of years since the menopause. In middle age these may be more relevant factors than chronological age in the interpretation of BMD results. There is an argument therefore for plotting results for pre- and postmenopausal women separately and interpreting values for postmenopausal women as a function of years after the menopause[27].

The T-score

The T-score is similar to the Z-score except that the mean and SD of the young-adult age group (20–35 years) is used as the reference range, regardless of the age of the patient whose BMD is being interpreted. T-scores compare a given subject with the sex and race adjusted expected maximum BMD achieved in life. The T-score is defined by the equation:

$$T\text{-score} = \frac{\text{Measured BMD} - \text{Young adult mean BMD}}{\text{Young adult standard deviation}}$$

A recent WHO technical report[28,29] advocated an interpretation of bone densitometry measurements based on T-score values in which subjects are divided into four categories:

(1) Normal: a value of BMD not more than 1 SD below the young-adult mean value ($T > -1.0$).

(2) Osteopenia: a BMD value that lies between 1 and 2.5 SD below the young-adult mean $(-1.0 > T > -2.5)$. Such individuals include those in whom the prevention of bone loss would be most useful.

(3) Osteoporosis: a BMD value more than 2.5 SD below the young-adult mean value $(T < -2.5)$.

(4) Established osteoporosis: a BMD value more than 2.5 SD below the young-adult mean value $(T < -2.5)$ in the presence of one or more fragility fractures.

The WHO definition of osteopenia and osteoporosis are useful because they bear an immediate relationship to the fracture threshold which is approximately 2 SD below the young normal mean $(T = -2)$[30]. In addition, T-score values are useful when interpreting the results of young adults and perimenopausal women because they indicate how the subject compares with her peers before the effects of age and the menopause. However, caution may be needed in the interpretation of T-score values in the older-age population when due to normal age-related bone loss even the mean BMD values may be below the −2.5 SD limit of the young-adult normal range. For older women over the age of 65–70 years the use of Z-scores is likely to be more appropriate. Further, some caution is necessary in younger women if therapeutic decisions are to be based on the present WHO criteria of osteopenia as a T-score of −1 will capture a high percentage of postmenopausal women, e.g. approximately 20% of women in their 60s[31].

Clinical indications for bone density measurements

Over the years many studies have identified factors that may affect bone-mass or fracture risk[32–34] and which may be considered as indicators for bone densitometry measurements. For most of these indications, however, the routine clinical use of BMD measurements is not justified since the correlations are either too weak or the results are unlikely to influence patient or clinician behaviour.

Table 1 Clinical indications for bone mass measurements

Menopausal women where result will influence treatment, e.g. with
  oestrogen replacement therapy
Oestrogen deficient women, e.g. early menopause, amenorrhoea or
  anorexia nervosa
Radiograph indicates osteopenia or vertebral deformity
Fracture after minor trauma
Steroid therapy, e.g. > 7 mg prednisolone/day
Diseases such as rheumatoid arthritis or primary hyperparathyroidism
  where result may influence treatment
To monitor response to treatment for osteoporosis

A number of clinical indications felt to justify bone densitometry
are listed in Table 1. These include scans of peri- and postmenopausal women where a low BMD result might influence the
decision to commence hormone replacement therapy, women who
are oestrogen deficient due to an early menopause, amenorrhoea or
anorexia, and patients who have suffered fractures after relatively
minor trauma, have been on long-term steroid therapy, or in whom
a recent radiograph suggests osteopenia.

The use of repeat BMD measurements to monitor the rate of bone
loss or the response of patients commencing treatment needs careful
consideration. The sensitivity of bone densitometry measurements
for these purposes is limited by the natural slow rates of loss and
the long-term precision of the technique as discussed above in relation to the characteristic follow-up time. This is the time required to
determine whether an individual has successfully responded to
treatment (i.e. BMD is no longer falling) or is still losing bone at the
average rate (–1.5%/year in the early postmenopausal years). It is
equally the time to distinguish whether an individual is losing at the
average rate or at twice that rate (i.e. could be considered as a fast
loser). For DXA of the lumbar spine this period is about 3 years[35].
Only larger rates of gain or loss can be detected in a shorter time
period, a factor that limits the value of repeating scans after too
short an interval.

REFERENCES

1. Blake, G.M., Tong, C.M. and Fogelman, I. (1991). Intersite comparison of the Hologic QDR-1000 dual energy X-ray bone densitometer. *Br. J. Radiol.*, **64**, 440–6
2. Lewis, M.K., Blake, G.M. and Fogelman, I. (1994). Patient dose in dual X-ray absorptiometry. *Osteoporosis Int.*, **4**, 11–15
3. Sorenson, J.A., Duke, P.R. and Smith, S.W. (1989). Stimulation studies of dual-energy X-ray absorptiometry. *Med. Phys.*, **16**, 75–80
4. Wahner, H.W. and Fogelman, I. (1994). *The Evaluation of Osteoporosis: Dual Energy X-ray Absorptiometry in Clinical Practice.* (London: Martin Dunitz)
5. Pommet, R., Chambellan, D., Reverchon, P., Pare, C., Lecluse, A. and Panissier, P. (1991). Array multidetector bone densitometer for supine lateral vertebral measurement in lateral projection. *Osteoporosis Int.*, **1**, 190
6. Steiger, P., von Stetten, E., Weiss, H. and Stein, J.A. (1991). Paired AP and lateral supine dual X-ray absorptiometry of the spine: initial results with a 32 detector system. *Osteoporosis Int.*, **1**, 190
7. Blake, G.M., Parker, J.C., Buxton, F.M.A. and Fogelman, I. (1993). Dual X-ray absorptiometry: a comparison between fan beam and pencil beam scans. *Br. J. Radiol.*, **66**, 902–6
8. Faulkner, K.G., Glüer, C.-C., Estillo, M. and Genant, H.K. (1993). Cross-calibration of DXA equipment: upgrading from a Hologic QDR-1000/W to a QDR-2000. *Calcif. Tissue Int.*, **52**, 79–84
9. Herd, R.J.M., Blake, G.M., Parker, J.C., Ryan, P.J. and Fogelman, I. (1993). Total body studies in normal British women using dual X-ray absorptiometry. *Br. J. Radiol.*, **66**, 303–8
10. Snead, D.B., Birge, S.J. and Kohrt, W.M. (1993). Age related differences in body composition by hydrodensitometry and dual-energy X-ray absorptiometry. *J. Appl. Physiol.*, **74**, 770–5
11. Richmond, B.J., Eberle R.W., Stulberg, B.N. and Deal, C.L. (1991). DEXA measurement of peri-prosthetic bone mineral density in total hip arthroplasty. *Osteoporosis Int.*, **1**, 191
12. Trevisan, C., Cherubini, R., Ulivieri, F.M., Gandolini, G.G., Randelli, G. and Ortolani, S. (1991). Dual energy X-ray absorptiometry in the evaluation of periprosthetic bone mineral status: analysis protocols and reproducibility. *Osteoporosis Int.*, **1**, 191
13. Jones, C.D., Laval-Jeantet, A.M., Laval-Jeantet, M.H. and Genant, H.K. (1987). Importance of measurement of spongious vertebral bone mineral density in the assessment of osteoporosis. *Bone*, **8**, 201–6

14. Larnach, T.A., Boyd, S.J., Smart, R.C., Butler, S.P., Rohl, P.G. and Diamond, T.H. (1992). Reproducibility of lateral spine scans using dual energy X-ray absorptiometry. *Calcif. Tissue Int.*, **51**, 255–8

15. Slosman, D.O., Rizzoli, R., Donath, A. and Bonjour, J.-Ph. (1990). Vertebral bone mineral density measured laterally by dual energy X-ray absorptiometry. *Osteoporosis Int.*, **1**, 23–9

16. Blake, G.M., Jagathesan, T., Herd, R.J.M. and Fogelman, I. (1994). Dual X-ray absorptiometry of the lumbar spine: the precision of paired anteriorposterior/lateral studies. *Br. J. Radiol.*, **67**, 624–30

17. Black, D.M., Cummings, S.R., Stone, K., Hudes, E., Palermo, L. and Streiger, P. (1991). A new approach to defining normal vertebral dimensions. *J. Bone Miner. Res.*, **6**, 883–92

18. Eastell, R., Cedel, S.L., Wahner, H.W., Riggs, B.L. and Melton, J.J. (1991). Classification of vertebral fractures. *J. Bone Miner. Res.*, **6**, 207–15

19. McCloskey, E.V., Spector, T.D., Eyres, K.S., Fern, E.D., O'Rourke, N., Vasikaran, S. and Kanis, J.A. (1993). The assessment of vertebral deformity: a method for use in population studies and clinical trials. *Osteoporosis Int.*, **3**, 138–47

20. Steiger, P., Cummings, S.R., Genant, H.K. and Weiss, H. (1994). Morphometric X-ray absorptiometry: correlation *in vivo* with morphometric radiography. *Osteoporosis Int.*, **4**, 238–44

21. Edmonston, S.J., Singer, K.P., Price, R.I. and Breidahl, P.D. (1993). Accuracy of lateral dual energy X-ray absorptiometry for the determination of bone mineral content in the thoracic and lumber spine: an *in vitro* study. *Br. J. Radiol.*, **66**, 309–13

22. Erikson, S., Isberg, B. and Lindgren, U. (1988). Vertebral bone mineral measurement using dual photon absorptiometry and computed tomography. *Acta Radiologica*, **29**, 89–94

23. Gotfredsen, A., Podenphant, J., Norgaard, H., Nilas, L., Nielsen, V.A. and Christiansen, C. (1988). Accuracy of lumbar spine bone mineral content by dual photon absorptiometry. *J. Nucl. Med.*, **29**, 248–54

24. Ho, C.P., Kim, R.W., Schaffler, M.B. and Sartoris, D.J. (1990). Accuracy of dual-energy radiographic absorptiometry of the lumbar spine: a cadaver study. *Radiology*, **176**, 171–3

25. Mazess, R., Collick, B., Trempe, J., Barden, H. and Hanson, J. (1989). Performance evaluation of a dual-energy X-ray bone densitometer. *Calcif. Tissue Int.*, **44**, 228–32

26. Ramalingam, T., Herd, R.J.M., Lees, B., Blake, G.M., Stevenson, J.G., Miller, C.G. and Fogelman, I. (1993). A comparison of three commercial bone ultrasound scanners. *Calcif. Tissue Int.*, **52**, 170

27. Ryan, P.J., Blake, G.M. and Fogelman, I. (1992). Postmenopausal screening for osteopenia. *Br. J. Rheumatol.*, **31**, 823–8

28. WHO Technical Report Series 843 (1994). *Assessment of fracture risk and its application to screening for postmenopausal osteoporosis.* (Geneva: World Health Organization)

29. Kanis, J.A., Melton, L.J., Christiansen, C., Johnston, C.C. and Khaltaev, N. (1994). The diagnosis of osteoporosis. *J. Bone Miner. Res.*, **9**, 1137–41

30. Ryan, P.J., Blake, G.M. and Fogelman, I. (1992). Fracture thresholds in osteoporosis: implications for hormone replacement therapy. *Ann. Rheum. Dis.*, **51**, 1063–5

31. Melton, L.J. (1995). How many women have osteoporosis now? *J. Bone Miner. Res.*, **10**, 175–7

32. Aloia, J.F., Cohn, S.H., Vaswani, A., Yeh, J.K., Yuen, K. and Ellis, K. (1985). Risk factors for postmenopausal osteoporosis. *Am. J. Med.*, **78**, 95–100

33. Elders, P.J.M., Netelenbos, J.C., Lips, P., Khoe, E., van Ginkel, F.G., Hulshof, K.F. and van der Stelt, P.F. (1989). Perimenopausal bone mass and risk factors. *Bone Miner.*, **7**, 289–99

34. Slemenda, C.W., Hui, S.L., Longcope, C., Wellman, H. and Johnston, C.C. (1990). Predictors of bone mass in perimenopausal women. *Ann. Intern. Med.*, **112**, 96–101

35. Glüer, C.-C., Blunt, B., Engelke, M. *et al.* (1994). Characteristic follow-up time: a new concept for standardized characterization of a technique's ability to monitor longitudinal changes. *Bone Miner.*, **25**, (Suppl. 2), S40

61

5

Bone morphology: quality, quantity and strength

J.E. Compston

INTRODUCTION

Oestrogen deficiency plays a central role in the development of postmenopausal osteoporosis and the beneficial effects of oestrogen replacement on bone mass have been well established[1-9]. However, the mechanisms by which oestrogen depletion and repletion affect bone remodelling and structure remain only partially defined; in particular, the evolution of structural disruption in cancellous bone associated with oestrogen deficiency and the potential for conventional hormone replacement therapy to produce anabolic effects have not been resolved.

BONE REMODELLING

Bone remodelling occurs at discrete sites on the cancellous bone surface and around Haversian systems in cortical bone and is the process by which the mechanical integrity of the skeleton is maintained in adult humans (Figure 1). A quantum of bone is removed by osteoclasts and subsequently replaced, within the cavity so formed, by osteoblasts[10]. Before remodelling can occur, preparation of the quiescent surface is required, a process involving retraction of lining cells and removal of the thin, collagen-containing membrane

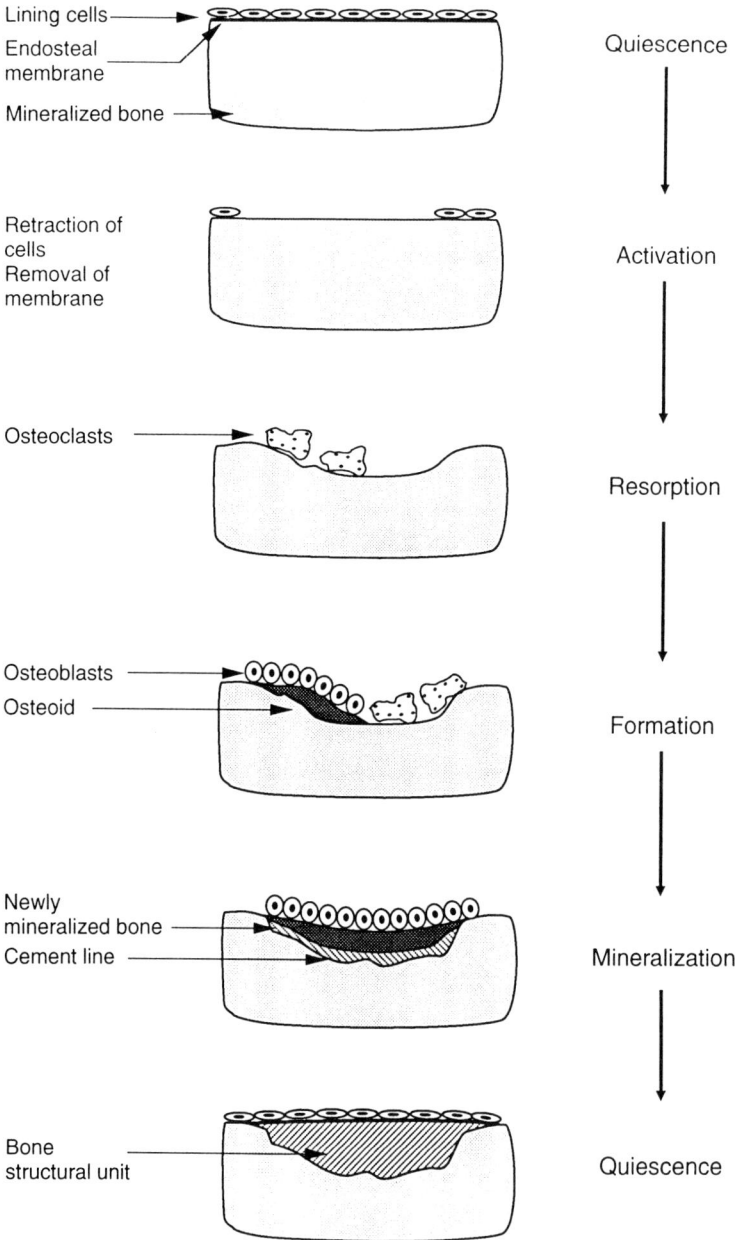

Lining cells

Endosteal membrane

Mineralized bone

Quiescence

Retraction of cells
Removal of membrane

Activation

Osteoclasts

Resorption

Osteoblasts

Osteoid

Formation

Newly mineralized bone

Cement line

Mineralization

Bone structural unit

Quiescence

Figure 1 Diagram to illustrate bone remodelling in cancellous bone

covering the bone surface. This is known as activation and involves the production, by bone cells, of proteolytic enzymes including metalloproteinases.

In normal adult human bone the temporal sequence of events in remodelling is always that of resorption followed by formation, a phenomenon referred to as coupling. In young adults, the amounts of bone resorbed and formed within individual units are similar, maintaining a state of remodelling balance. The activation frequency reflects the number of new remodelling units activated anywhere on the bone surface within a given time. The total time for one remodelling unit to undergo activation, resorption and formation is in the order of 3 to 6 months, most of this time being occupied by matrix formation and mineralization. Once the remodelling unit has been completed it is known as a bone structural unit.

The regulation of bone remodelling is complex and involves mechanical stimuli[11], systemic hormones and a variety of locally produced cytokines and growth factors[12] (Figure 2). Mechanical loading is believed to stimulate osteogenesis via effects on the osteocytes, which are embedded in the bone matrix and communicate with each other and with lining cells on the bone surface. The precise mechanisms by which these effects are mediated have not been defined but osteocytic activation by mechanical strains results in the production of a cascade of chemical messengers including prostaglandins, nitric oxide, glucose-6-phosphate dehydrogenase and insulin-like growth factors. Many systemic hormones affect bone remodelling (Table 1); they are believed to exert their effects, at least in part, via the production of locally produced growth factors. These cytokines and growth factors, which are produced by bone cells and cells in the bone micro-environment act in an autocrine or paracrine manner to regulate the proliferation and differentiation of bone cell precursors and, to a lesser extent, the activity of mature osteoclasts and osteoblasts (Table 2)[13].

MECHANISMS OF BONE LOSS IN OSTEOPOROSIS

Bone loss may occur by two basic mechanisms at the cellular level[14]. Quantitatively the most important is an increase in activation

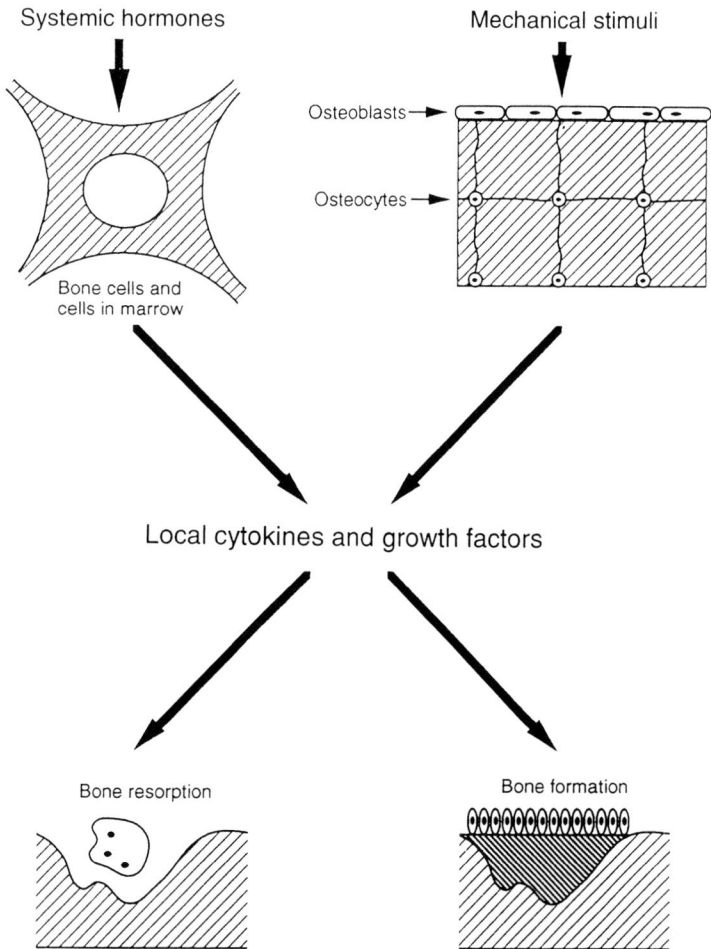

Figure 2 Factors involved in the regulation of bone remodelling. From Compston[71] with permission

frequency (increased bone turnover), which creates a greater number of resorption cavities on the bone surface at any given time; however, provided that remodelling balance is maintained, bone loss can be reversed if activation frequency is reduced. Second, a negative remodelling balance due to the resorption of a larger amount of bone within the remodelling unit (increased erosion depth) and/or formation of a smaller amount will result in bone

Table 1 Systemic hormones which affect bone remodelling

Parathyroid hormone
1,25-dihydroxyvitamin D3
Calcitonin
Thyroxine
Oestrogen
Androgens
Growth hormone
Glucocorticoids

Table 2 Cytokines and growth factors affecting bone

Stimulators of bone resorption
    Interleukins -1, 6, 8, 11 (IL-1, 6, 8, 11)
    Tumour necrosis factors (TNFs)
    Epidermal growth factor (EGF)
    Platelet-derived growth factor (PDGF)
    Fibroblast growth factors (FGFs)
    Leukaemia inhibitory factor (LIF)
    Macrophage colony stimulating factor (M-CSF)
    Granulocyte/macrophage colony stimulating factor (GM-CSF)
Inhibitors of bone resorption
    Interferon-γ (IFNγ)
    Interleukin-4 (IL-4)
Stimulators of bone formation
    Insulin-like growth factors (IGFs)
    Transforming growth factor-β (TGFβ)
    Fibroblast growth factors (FGFs)
    Platelet-derived growth factors (PDGFs)
    Bone morphogenetic proteins (BMPs)

loss, the magnitude of which will depend both on the degree of imbalance and the activation frequency. The combination of increased activation frequency and remodelling imbalance results in rapid bone loss, a component of which is irreversible.

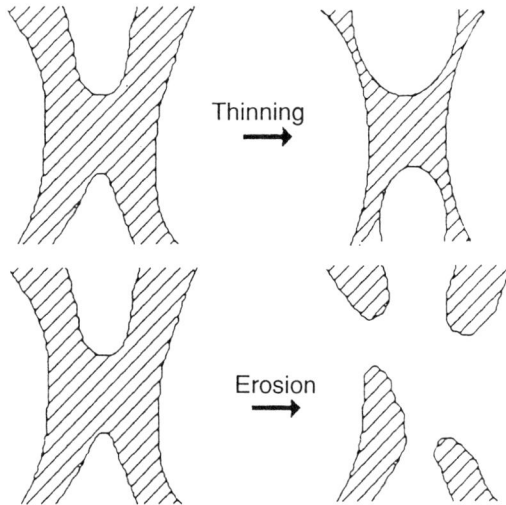

Figure 3 Structural mechanisms of cancellous bone loss. From Compston[72] with permission

BONE ARCHITECTURE

The changes in bone remodelling which underlie bone loss are responsible for the associated alterations in cancellous and cortical bone architecture[15]. An increase in activation frequency and/or increased erosion depth of individual remodelling units will predispose to trabecular penetration and erosion (Figure 3), whereas trabecular thinning, due to reduced bone formation, will be associated with better preservation of bone architecture although the risk of penetration by a resorption cavity of normal depth increases progressively as trabecular thickness decreases.

These structural changes have important mechanical and therapeutic implications. Trabecular penetration and erosion result in greater loss of bone strength for any given bone mass than trabecular thinning; moreover, it is unlikely that any treatment can restore bone structure, once this has been disrupted, whereas the ability of drugs to thicken existing trabeculae is well documented[16]. The severe disruption of cancellous bone architecture in postmenopausal osteoporosis emphasizes the importance of early intervention, before irreversible changes have occurred.

Cortical bone is also an important determinant of bone strength and fracture risk. Postmenopausal bone loss is associated with thinning of the cortex, mainly as a result of endocortical changes which result in 'trabecularization' of the cortex and consequent loss of mechanical strength, an effect which is not wholly compensated for by the periosteal apposition of bone which occurs with increasing age and results in an increase in the transverse diameter of bones[17].

HISTOMORPHOMETRIC ASSESSMENT OF BONE REMODELLING AND STRUCTURE

The measurement of static and dynamic indices of bone resorption and formation in histological sections of bone enables quantitative assessment of the contribution made by alterations in bone turnover and remodelling imbalance to changes in bone mass in untreated and treated osteoporosis[14]. Using the technique of double tetracycline labelling, the bone formation rate at tissue level can be measured and activation frequency and bone turnover calculated[18]. Tetracycline is given to the patient in two, time-spaced doses prior to the biopsy and is taken up at actively forming bone surfaces (Figure 4); since no equivalent marker exists for activation or bone resorption, the calculation of activation frequency and resorption rates is performed using the bone formation rate, based on the assumptions that bone remodelling is in a steady state and that resorption and formation are coupled, neither of which may be tenable in disease states.

The assessment of remodelling balance requires measurement both of the amount of bone resorbed and formed within each remodelling unit. Measurement of the erosion depth can be achieved by computerized or manual reconstruction of the eroded bone surface[19], although identification of resorption cavities can be difficult and determination of those in which resorption has been completed is problematic. The amount of bone formed within remodelling units, known as the wall width, can be measured after identification of bone structural units under polarized light (Figure 5) or by conventional light microscopy using staining techniques to identify the

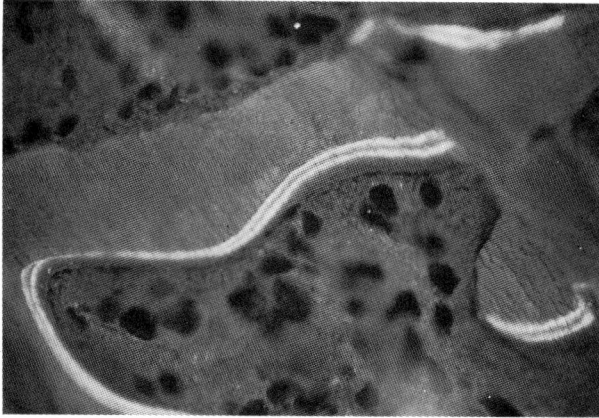

Figure 4 Tetracycline fluorescence at the actively mineralizing surfaces of human cancellous bone, viewed by fluorescence microscopy. Two separate lines, representing the time-spaced labels, can be clearly seen

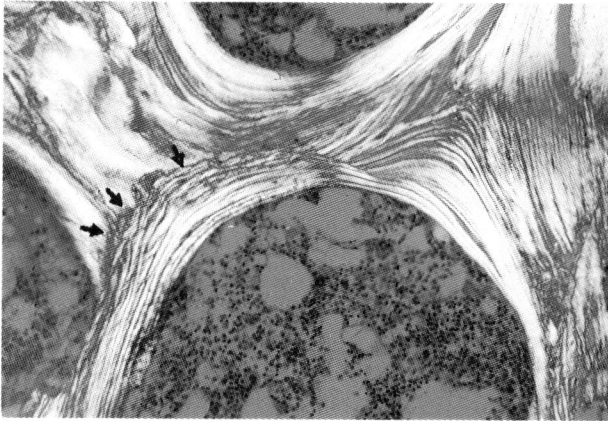

Figure 5 A completed bone structural unit viewed by polarized light microscopy. The arrow indicates the cement line

cement line, which represents the base of the original resorption cavity[20].

A number of techniques have been described for the quantitative assessment of cancellous bone structure[21]. Trabecular width, separation and number can be measured directly or calculated; more sophisticated methods include strut analysis, trabecular bone pattern factor and marrow star volume. The method of strut analysis is based on the definition of nodes and termini in two-dimensional sections and the topological classification of trabeculae or struts[22]. Trabecular bone pattern factor is based on the principle that concave surfaces indicate structural connectedness whilst the reverse is true for convex surfaces. Measurement of the bone area and perimeter before and after computer-simulated dilatation results in an increase of bone perimeter of convex structures and a decrease of concave ones[23]. Other methods include the marrow star volume, fractal analysis and three-dimensional approaches using reconstruction of serial sections or microcomputed tomography.

THE RELATIONSHIP BETWEEN BONE MASS, ARCHITECTURE AND FRACTURE RISK

Bone mass is a major determinant of bone strength and fracture risk[24]. Prospective studies have shown an increasing gradient of fracture risk with decreasing bone density, a decrease of one standard deviation in the latter being associated with a two- to three-fold increase in fracture risk[25–28]. This relationship, which is similar to that observed between hypertension and stroke or serum lipid profile and coronary artery disease, is seen for bone density at all sites commonly assessed and for all types of fragility fracture.

The extent to which alterations in bone architecture contribute to bone fragility, independent of changes in bone mass, is uncertain. The important contribution of cortical bone to compressive strength and the tendency for changes in cancellous bone mass and structure to occur simultaneously suggest that bone densitometry is a reasonable surrogate for bone strength, particularly if both cortical and cancellous bone are included.

Nonetheless, some lines of evidence support an independent role for bone architecture as a determinant of bone strength. Some studies have demonstrated greater disruption of cancellous bone structure in women with osteoporotic fracture than in age-matched control subjects with similar bone mass[29,30], although this finding has not been universal[31]. In addition, the evidence that one or more prevalent or past fragility fractures substantially increases subsequent

Normal turnover   Remodelling balance

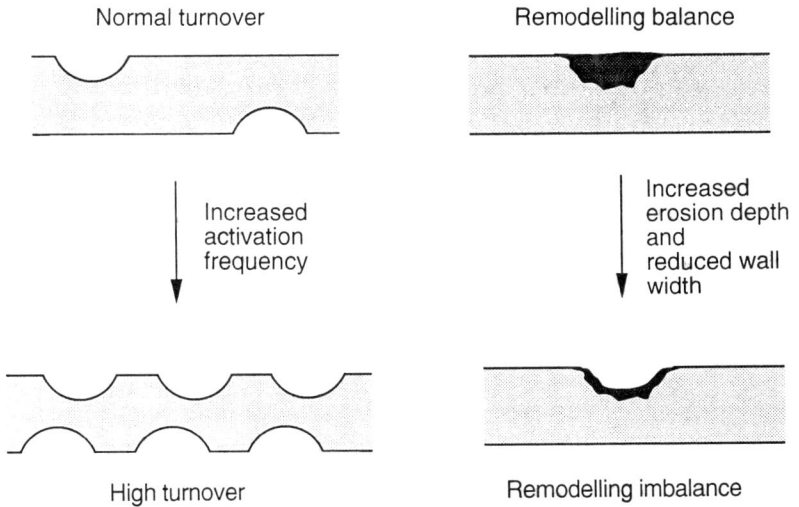

Increased activation frequency

Increased erosion depth and reduced wall width

High turnover   Remodelling imbalance

Figure 6 Diagram to illustrate the pathophysiology of postmenopausal bone loss

fracture risk, regardless of bone mass, indicates that bone architecture may contribute independently to bone strength[32]. The observation that very small changes in cancellous microstructure can have significant mechanical implications further supports this contention.

PATHOPHYSIOLOGY OF MENOPAUSAL BONE LOSS

There is considerable evidence from balance studies and biochemical data that increased bone turnover plays a major role in the pathogenesis of menopausal bone loss[33] (Figure 6). Indices of bone resorption, such as urinary hydroxyproline and collagen cross-link excretion and serum tartrate acid phosphatase concentration increase rapidly after oophorectomy, followed by a slower rise in markers of bone formation such as serum alkaline phosphatase and osteocalcin[34]. These changes are maximal around 12 months after oophorectomy and may take up to 10 years to normalize in untreated women; conversely, oestrogen administration at the time of or soon after oophorectomy abolishes these changes.

Histomorphometric data are relatively sparse but show a less clear-cut picture, with considerable heterogeneity in indices of bone turnover in women with postmenopausal osteoporosis[35–37]. This may reflect a number of factors, including measurement variance, skeletal heterogeneity of disease and intermittency of changes in remodelling. Furthermore, the increase in bone remodelling may be relatively transient and occur only in the early stages of the menopause. A more consistent finding in postmenopausal osteoporosis is remodelling imbalance, associated with a reduction in the amount of bone formed within each remodelling unit[38–40]. This may indicate the presence of osteoblast dysfunction, although an alternative explanation is that women who develop osteoporosis have a lower peak bone mass and smaller bone structural units than those who are unaffected. Increased erosion depth due to increased osteoclastic activity may also contribute to remodelling imbalance, although direct evidence for such an effect in humans is lacking.

The mechanisms by which oestrogen affects bone remodelling have not been clearly defined. Both osteoclastic and osteoblastic cells possess oestrogen receptors[41–43], although their density is less than in classic target cells. Direct effects of oestrogen on osteoblasts and osteoclasts in humans have not been demonstrated, but there is considerable evidence that oestrogen modulates the production, by mononuclear cells in the bone micro-environment, of several bone-active cytokines including interleukin-1, tumour necrosis factor α and granulocyte-macrophage colony stimulating factor[44,45]. Interleukin-6, a stimulator of osteoclastogenesis, may also be implicated[46]. Although oestrogen-induced stimulation of growth factors with the potential to increase bone formation has been reported in cell culture[47], the significance of these findings *in vivo* is uncertain.

EFFECTS OF ACUTE OESTROGEN DEFICIENCY ON BONE REMODELLING AND STRUCTURE IN PREMENOPAUSAL WOMEN

The use of gonadotrophin releasing hormone (GnRH) analogues in the treatment of endometriosis and other gynaecological disorders in premenopausal women provides a unique model for investigation of

Table 3 Bone remodelling and structure before and after 6 months treatment with gonadotrophin releasing hormone analogues

	Pretreatment	*Post-treatment*
Erosion depth (µm)	23.1 ± 3.8	21.3 ± 3.2
Wall width (µm)	39.2 ± 7.1	35.5 ± 4.1
Bone formation rate ($\mu m^2/\mu m/day$)	0.049 ± 0.036	0.062 ± 0.054
Activation frequency (/year)	0.46 ± 0.38	0.67 ± 0.63
Node/terminus ratio	1.3 ± 0.8	0.7 ± 0.6*
Trabecular bone pattern factor (mm^{-1})	0.19 ± 1.7	1.01 ± 1.3*

*$p < 0.05$

the skeletal effects of acute oestrogen deficiency. These analogues produce an initial stimulation of the pituitary–ovarian axis followed by rapid and severe oestrogen deficiency. Densitometric studies have demonstrated rapid bone loss, particularly in the spine, after 6 months treatment with these drugs[48–53]; although bone mass is partially or fully restored after therapy is withdrawn, the magnitude of bone loss suggests that irreversible changes may occur in cancellous bone structure, exposing these women to a higher risk of fracture in later years.

The effects of GnRH agonists on bone remodelling and structure have recently been reported in a group of women undergoing treatment for endometriosis[54]. Iliac crest biopsies were obtained before and 6 months after treatment; most women received unopposed GnRH analogue therapy although some were also given add-back therapy in the form of tibolone (Livial®). In those receiving GnRH analogue therapy alone there was an increase in bone formation rate and activation frequency, both indices of bone turnover, with a small reduction in the amount of bone resorbed and formed within individual remodelling units (erosion depth and wall width respectively; Table 3). Despite these relatively small changes in indices of bone remodelling, however, there was qualitative and quantitative evidence of severe disruption of iliac crest cancellous-bone structure in these women (Figure 7), with evidence of widespread trabecular penetra-

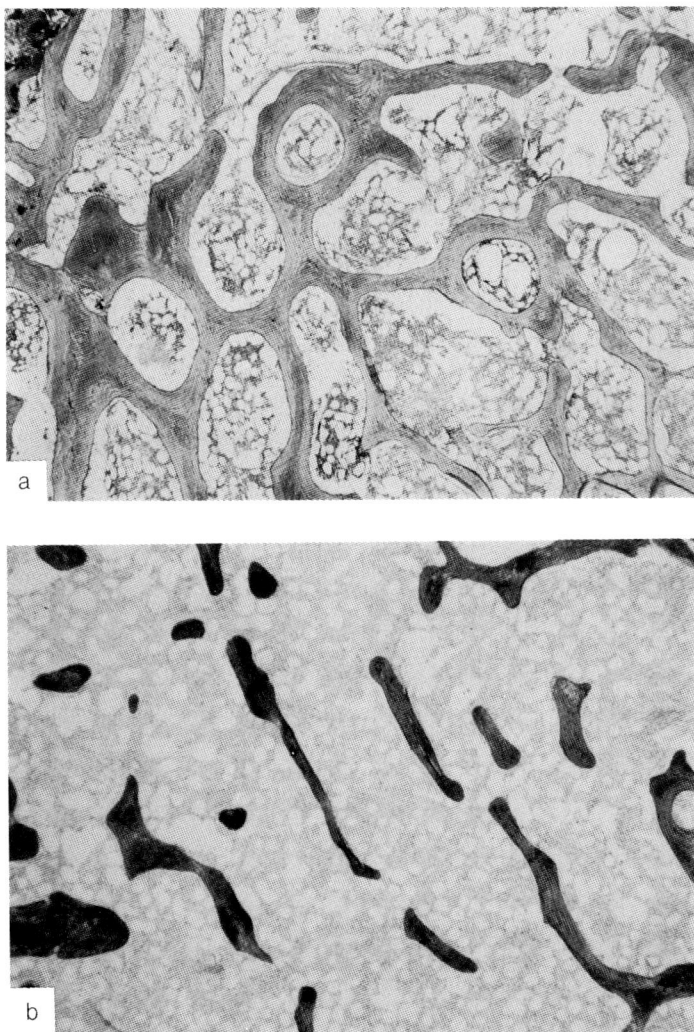

Figure 7 Iliac crest cancellous bone from a 28-year-old woman with endo-metriosis before (a) and after (b) 6 months GnRH analogue therapy

tion and erosion resulting in reduced trabecular connectedness. These observations were confirmed by quantitative structural analysis (Table 3), which demonstrated a significant decrease in the node to terminus ratio and increase in trabecular bone pattern factor.

These data demonstrate that acute oestrogen deficiency, induced by GnRH analogues, results in significant disruption of cancellous bone structure which is unlikely to be reversible and may be associated with increased fracture risk in later life. The structural changes observed cannot be explained on the basis of the relatively small alterations in bone turnover and remodelling balance and indicate that different pathophysiological mechanisms operate during the early stages of oestrogen deficiency. The degree of structural disruption suggests that increased erosion depth is likely to play a major role in bone loss and the associated trabecular penetration; the early and transient nature of this effect, together with the inability to measure resorption cavities which have resulted in trabecular penetration, may explain the lack of evidence for an increase in erosion depth in biopsies obtained at 6 months. In those women receiving both GnRH analogues and tibolone, indices of bone remodelling and structure were very similar in pre- and post-treatment biopsies. Although the number of women in this group was too small to enable definite conclusions to be drawn, the results obtained suggest that tibolone reduces or reverses the adverse effects of GnRH analogues on bone; other possible approaches to add-back therapy include the use of progestogens or combined oestrogen/progestogens[55-57].

THE EFFECTS OF LONG-TERM HORMONE REPLACEMENT THERAPY ON BONE REMODELLING AND STRUCTURE

Despite the widespread use of hormone replacement therapy to prevent bone loss and reduce fracture risk its effects on bone remodelling and structure are incompletely understood. Measurement of biochemical markers of bone turnover indicates that the administration of hormone replacement therapy is associated with a reduction in bone turnover, a conclusion supported by histomorphometric assessment of activation frequency and bone formation rate[58-60]. Thus the increase in bone turnover which occurs during the menopause appears to be causally related to oestrogen deficiency and can be completely reversed by oestrogen replacement.

The other component of menopausal bone loss, namely remodelling imbalance, is less well studied. Biochemical markers of bone resorption and formation are insufficiently sensitive to reflect changes in remodelling balance, which can only be assessed by histomorphometric techniques. An age-related decrease in the wall width, reflecting the amount of bone formed within individual bone remodelling units, has been shown in both men and women and begins around the fifth decade of life[38,61] but it is unclear whether, in women, this is related to oestrogen deficiency and can be corrected by hormone replacement. Erosion depth and wall width before and after oestrogen treatment have only been assessed in two studies. Steiniche and colleagues[58] reported no significant change in erosion depth or wall width in ten women with postmenopausal osteoporosis treated with hormone replacement therapy for 1 year. More recently, we have studied 22 postmenopausal women with osteoporosis before and after 2 years hormone replacement therapy[62]. Consistent trends were seen towards a reduction in resorption cavity size, with a quantitatively similar reduction in wall width; these data thus provide no evidence that conventional hormone replacement therapy has anabolic effects at the level of the bone remodelling unit.

Small increases in bone mass in women treated with hormone replacement therapy have been demonstrated by bone densitometry[4,5,63–65]; these changes have generally been of the order of 1–2%/year although larger increases have been reported, particularly in women treated with oestradiol implants[66]. These increments in bone mass are unlikely to reflect anabolic skeletal effects and can be fully accounted for by the reduction in bone turnover induced by oestrogen replacement and the corresponding in-filling of the remodelling space. Indeed, in view of the relatively low bone turnover induced by oestrogen therapy, any anabolic effect at the level of the individual bone remodelling unit (i.e. a greater amount of bone formed than resorbed) would be unlikely to have a significant impact on bone mass. High doses of oestrogen have been shown to produce anabolic effects in rat bone[67], but this results from *de novo* bone formation in a modelling species and may not be relevant to adult humans.

The potential for pharmacological doses of oestrogen to produce anabolic skeletal effects, although not yet demonstrated in humans, has prompted the suggestion that high doses of selective oestrogen agonists such as droloxifene and raloxifene might also be anabolic and thus prove more effective than conventional hormone replacement therapy. This possibility is attractive but remains unproven; in addition, drug-induced *de novo* bone formation may result in the production of mechanically inferior bone, at least until newly-formed woven bone is remodelled. An example of this is provided by high-dose sodium fluoride therapy, which despite producing impressive increases in bone mass may be associated with reduced bone strength and increased fracture risk. Finally, whilst the development of bone anabolic drugs is conceptually attractive, the benefits of antiresorptive drugs should not be underestimated, even in elderly subjects with low bone mass; thus significant reductions in fracture risk were demonstrated in very elderly women after only 18 months treatment with calcium and vitamin D[68], a finding which may be explained by the continuation of bone loss throughout life[69] and the increasing importance of bone mass as a determinant of fracture risk with age[70].

REFERENCES

1. Albright, F., Smith, P.H. and Richardson, A.M. (1941). Postmenopausal osteoporosis. *J. Am. Med. Assoc.*, **116**, 2465–74
2. Compston, J.E. (1992). HRT and osteoporosis. *Br. Med. Bull.*, **48**, 309–44
3. Lindsay, R., Hart, D.M., Forrest, C. and Baird, C (1980). Prevention of spinal osteoporosis in oophorectomised women. *Lancet*, **2**, 1151–3
4. Christiansen, C., Christensen, M.S., McNair, P.L., Hagen, C., Stocklund, K.E. and Transbol, I. (1980). Prevention of early postmenopausal bone loss: conducted 2-year study in 315 normal females. *Eur. J. Clin. Invest.*, **10**, 273–9
5. Ettinger, B., Genant, H.K. and Cann, C.E. (1985). Long-term oestrogen replacement therapy prevents bone loss and fractures. *Ann. Intern. Med.*, **102**, 319–24
6. Hutchinson, A., Polansky, S.M. and Feinstein, A.R. (1979). Post-menopausal estrogens protect against fractures of the hip and distal radius: a case control study. *Lancet*, **2**, 705–9
7. Weiss, N.S., Ure, C.L., Ballard, J.H., Williams, A.R. and Daling, J.R. (1980). Decreased risk of fractures of the hip and lower forearm with postmenopausal use of estrogens. *N. Engl. J. Med.*, **303**, 1195–8

8.   Paganini-Hill, A., Ross, R.K., Gerkins, V.R., Henderson, B.E., Arthur, M. and Mack, T.M. (1981). Menopausal estrogen therapy and hip fractures. *Ann. Intern. Med.*, **95**, 28–31

9.   Kiel, D.P., Felson, D.T., Anderson, J.J., Wilson, P.W.F. and Moskowitz, M.A. (1987). Hip fracture and the use of estrogens in postmenopausal women: the Framingham study. *N. Engl. J. Med.*, **317**, 1169–74

10. Parfitt, A.M. (1984). The cellular basis of bone remodelling. The quantum concept re-examined in light of recent advances in cell biology of bone. *Calcif. Tissue Int.*, **36**, S37–45

11. Lanyon, L.E. (1992). The success and failure of the adaptive response to functional load-bearing in averting vertebral fracture. *Bone*, **13** (Suppl. 2), S17–21

12. Russell, R.G.G. (1989). The physiological regulation of bone metabolism. In Ring, E.F.J. Evans, W.D. and Dixon, A.S. (eds.) *Osteoporosis and Bone Mineral Measurement*, pp. 147–76. (York, England: IPSM)

13. MacDonald, B.R. and Gowen, M. (1992). Cytokines and bone. *Br. J. Rheumatol.*, **31**, 149–55

14. Compston, J.E. and Croucher, P.I. (1991). Histomorphometric assessment of trabecular bone remodelling in osteoporosis. *Bone Miner.*, **14**, 91–102

15. Compston, J.E., Mellish, R.W.E., Croucher, P.I., Newcombe, R. and Garrahan, N.J. (1989). Structural mechanisms of trabecular bone loss in man. *Bone Miner.*, **6**, 339–50

16. Briancon, D. and Meunier, P.J. (1981). Treatment of osteoporosis with fluoride, calcium and vitamin D. *Orthop. Clin. North Am.,*, **12**, 629–48

17. Compston, J.E. (1995). Bone mineral density: BMC, BMD or corrected BMD? *Bone*, **16**, 5–7

18. Frost, H.M. (1969). Tetracycline-based histological analysis of bone remodelling. *Calcif. Tissue Int.*, **3**, 211–37

19. Garrahan, N.J., Croucher, P.I. and Compston, J.E. (1990). A computerised technique for the quantitative assessment of resorption cavities in trabecular bone. *Bone*, **11**, 241–6

20. Lips, P., Courpron, P. and Meunier, P.J. (1978). Mean wall thickness of trabecular bone packets in the human iliac crest: changes with age. *Calcif. Tissue Res.* , **26**, 13–17

21. Compston, J.E. (1994). Connectivity of cancellous bone: assessment and mechanical implications. *Bone*, **15**, 463–6

22. Garrahan, N.J., Mellish, R.W.E. and Compston, J.E. (1986). A new method for the two-dimensional analysis of bone structure in human iliac crest biopsies. *J. Microsc.*, **142**, 341–9

23. Hahn, M., Vogel, M., Pompesius-Kempa, M. and Delling, G. (1992). Trabecular bone pattern factor – a new parameter for simple quantification of bone microarchitecture. *Bone*, **13**, 327–30

24. Hayes, W.C. and Gerhart, T.N. (1985). Biomechanics of bone: applications for assessment of bone strength. In Peck, W.A. (ed.) *Bone and Mineral Research 3*, pp. 259–94. (Amsterdam: Elsevier)
25. Wasnich, R.D., Ross, P.D., Heilbrun, L.K. and Vogel, J.M. (1985). Prediction of postmenopausal fracture risk with bone mineral measurements. *Am. J. Obstet. Gynecol.*, **153**, 745–51
26. Hui, S.L., Slemenda, C.W. and Johnston, C.C. (1988). Age and bone mass as predictors of fracture in a prospective study. *J. Clin. Invest.*, **81**, 1804–9
27. Gärdsell, P., Johnell, O. and Nilsson, B. (1989). Predicting fractures in women by using forearm bone densitometry. *Calcif. Tissue Int.*, **44**, 235–42
28. Cummings, S.R., Black, D.M., Nevitt, M.C., Browner, W., Cauley, J., Ensrud, K., Genant, H.K., Palermo, L., Scott, J. and Vogt, T.M. (1993). Bone density at various sites for prediction of hip fractures. *Lancet*, **341**, 72–5
29. Kleerekoper, M., Villanueva, A.R., Stanciu, J., Rao, D.S. and Parfitt, A.M. (1985). The role of three dimensional trabecular microstructure in the pathogenesis of vertebral compression fractures. *Calcif. Tissue Int.*, **37**, 594–7
30. Recker, R.R., Smith, R.T. and Kimmel, D.B. (1992). Loss of trabecular connectivity in osteoporosis demonstrated with independent methods. *Bone*, **13**, A28
31. Croucher, P.I., Garrahan, N.J. and Compston, J.E. (1994). Structural mechanisms of trabecular bone loss in primary osteoporosis: specific disease mechanism or early ageing? *Bone Miner.*, **25**, 111–21
32. Ross, P.D., Davis, J.W., Epstein, R.S. and Wasnich, R.D. (1991). Pre-existing fractures and bone mass predict vertebral fracture incidence in women. *Ann. Intern. Med.*, **114**, 919–23
33. Heaney, R.P., Recker, R.R. and Saville, P.D. (1978). Menopausal changes in calcium balance performance. *J. Lab. Clin. Med.*, **92**, 953–63
34. Stepan, J.J., Pospichal, J., Presl, J. and Pacovsky, V. (1987). Bone loss and biochemical indices of bone remodelling in surgically induced postmenopausal women. *Bone*, **8**, 279–84
35. Whyte, P.M., Bergfeld, M.A., Murphy, W.A., Avioli, L.V. and Teitelbaum, S.L. (1982). Post-menopausal osteoporosis. A heterogenous disorder as assessed by histomorphometric analysis of iliac crest bone from untreated patients. *Am. J. Med.*, **72**, 192–202
36. Meunier, P.J., Courpron, P., Edouard, C., Alexandre, C., Bressot, C., Lips, P. and Boyce, B.F. (1979). Bone histomorphometry in

osteoporotic states. In Barzel, U.S. (ed.) *Osteoporosis 11*, pp. 27–47. (New York: Grune and Stratton)

37. Eriksen, E.F., Hodgson, S.F., Eastell, R., Cedel, S.L., O'Fallon, W.M. and Riggs, B.L. (1990). Cancellous bone remodelling in type I (postmenopausal) osteoporosis: quantitative assessment of rates of formation, resorption and bone loss at tissue and cellular levels. *J. Bone Miner. Res.*, **5**, 311–19

38. Darby, A.J. and Meunier, P.J. (1981). Mean wall thickness and formation periods of trabecular bone packets in idiopathic osteoporosis. *Calcif. Tissue Int*, **33**, 199–204

39. Garcia-Carasco, M., De Vernejoul, M.C., Sterkers, Y., Morieux, C., Kuntz, D. and Miravet, L. (1989). Decreased bone formation in osteoporotic patients compared to age-matched controls. *Calcif. Tissue Int.*, **44**, 173–5

40. Arlot, M., Edouard, C., Meunier, P.J., Neer, R.M. and Reeve, J. (1984). Impaired osteoblast function in osteoporosis: comparison between calcium balance and dynamic histomorphometry. *Br. Med. J.*, **289**, 517–20

41. Eriksen, E.F., Colvard, D.S., Berg, N.J., Graham, M.L., Mann, K.G., Spelsberg, T.C. and Riggs, B.L. (1988). Evidence of estrogen receptors in normal human osteoblast-like cells. *Science*, **241**, 84–6

42. Komm, B.S., Terpening, C.M., Benz, D.J., Graeme, K.A., Gallegos, A., Kork, M., Greene, G.L., O'Malley, B.W. and Haussler, M.R. (1988). Estrogen binding, receptor mRNA and biologic response in osteoblast-like osteosarcoma cells. *Science*, **241**, 81–4

43. Oursler, M.J., Pyfferoen, J., Osdoby, P., Riggs, B.L. and Spelsberg, T.C (1990). Osteoclasts express mRNA for estrogen receptor. *J. Bone Miner. Res.*, **5**, 517

44. Pacifici, R., Brown, C., Puscheck, E., Friedrich, E., Slatopolsky, E., Maggio, D., McCracken, R. and Avioli, L. (1991). Effect of surgical menopause and estrogen replacement on cytokine release from human blood mononuclear cells. *Proc. Natl. Acad. Sci. USA*, **88**, 5134–8

45. Ralston, S.H., Russell, R.G.G. and Gowen, M. (1990). Estrogen inhibits release of tumour necrosis factor from peripheral blood mononuclear cells in menopausal women. *J. Bone Miner. Res.*, **5**, 983–8

46. Jilka, R.L., Hangoc, G., Girasole, G., Passeri, G., Williams, D.C., Abrams, J.S., Boyce, B., Broxmeyer, H. and Manolagas, S. (1992). Increased osteoclast development after estrogen loss: mediation by interleukin-6. *Science*, **257**, 88–91

47. Gray, T.K., Mohan, S., Linkhart, T.A. and Baylink, D.J. (1989). Estradiol stimulates *in vitro* the secretion of insulin-like growth factors by the clonal osteoblastic cell-line, UMR 106. *Biochem. Biophys. Res. Commun.*, **158**, 407–12

48. Matta, W.H., Shaw, R.W., Hesp, R. and Evans, R. (1988). Reversible trabecular bone density loss following induced hypo-oestrogenism with the GnRH analogue buserelin in premenopausal women. *Clin. Endocrinol.*, **29**, 45–51

49. Johansen, J.S., Riis, B.J., Hassager, C., Moen, M., Jacobson, J. and Christiansen, C. (1988). The effect of a gonadotrophin-releasing hormone agonist (naferelin) on bone metabolism. *J. Clin. Endocrinol. Metab.*, **67**, 701–6

50. Dawood, M.Y., Lewis, V. and Ramos, J. (1989). Cortical and trabecular bone mineral content in women with endometriosis: effect of gonadotrophin-releasing hormone agonist and danazol. *Fertil. Steril.*, **52**, 21–6

51. Jacobson, J.B. (1990). Effects of naferelin on bone density. *Am. J. Obstet. Gynecol.*, **162**, 589–92

52. Whitehouse, R.W., Adams, J.E., Bancroft, K., Vaughan-Williams, C.A. and Elstein, M. (1990). The effects of naferelin and danazol on vertebral trabecular bone mass in patients with endometriosis. *Clin. Endocrinol.*, **33**, 365–73

53. Rico, H., Arnanz, F., Revilla, M., Perera, S., Iritia, M., Villa, L.F. and Arribas, I. (1993). Total and regional bone mineral content in women treated with GnRH agonists. *Calcif. Tissue Int.*, **52**, 354–7

54. Compston, J.E., Yamaguchi, K., Croucher, P.I., Garrahan, N.J., Lindsay, P.C. and Shaw, R.W. (1995). The effects of gonadotrophin-releasing agonists on iliac crest cancellous bone structure in women with endometriosis. *Bone*, **16**, 261–7

55. Riis, B.J., Christiansen, C., Johansen, J.S. and Jacobson, J. (1990). Is it possible to prevent bone loss in young women treated with luteinizing hormone-releasing hormone agonists. *J. Clin. Endocrinol. Metab.*, **70**, 920–4

56. Eldred, J.M., Haynes, P.J. and Thomas, E.J. (1992). A randomised double-blind controlled trial of the effects on bone metabolism of the combination of naferelin acetate and norethisterone. *Clin. Endocrinol.*, **37**, 354–9

57. Surrey, E.S. and Judd, H.L. (1992). Reduction of vasomotor symptoms and bone mineral density loss with combined norethindrone and long-acting gonadotrophin-releasing hormone agonist therapy of symptomatic endometriosis: a prospective randomised trial. *J. Clin. Endocrinol. Metab.*, **75**, 558–63

58. Steiniche, T., Hasling, C., Charles, P., Eriksen, E.F., Mosekilde, L. and Melsen, F. (1989). A randomised study on the effects of oestrogen-gestagen or high dose oral calcium on trabecular bone remodelling in postmenopausal osteoporosis. *Bone*, **10**, 313–20

59. Lufkin, E.G., Wahner, H.W., O'Fallon, W.M., Hodgson, S.F., Kotowicz, M.A., Lane, A.W., Judd, H.L., Caplan, R.H. and Riggs, B.L. (1992).

Treatment of postmenopausal osteoporosis with transdermal estrogen. *Ann. Intern. Med.*, **117**, 1–9

60. Holland, E.F., Chow, J.W.M., Studd, J.W.W., Leather, A.T. and Chambers, T.J. (1994). Histomorphometric changes in the skeleton of postmenopausal women with low bone mineral density treated with percutaneous implants. *Obstet. Gynecol.*, **83**, 387–91

61. Vedi, S., Compston, J.E., Webb, A. and Tighe, J.R. (1984). Histomorphometric analysis of bone biopsies from the iliac crest of normal British subjects. *Metab. Bone Dis. Rel. Res.*, **4**, 231–6

62. Vedi, S. and Compston, J.E. (1995). Effects of long-term hormone replacement therapy on bone remodelling in postmenopausal women. *Bone*, **17**, 323

63. Christiansen, C. and Riis, B.J. (1990). 17β-estradiol and continuous norethisterone: a unique treatment for established osteoporosis in elderly women. *J. Clin. Endocrinol. Metab.*, **71**, 836–41

64. Stevenson, J.C., Cust, M.P., Gangar, K.F., Hillard, T.C., Lees, B. and Whitehead, M.I. (1990). Effects of transdermal versus oral hormone replacement therapy on bone density in spine and proximal femur in postmenopausal women. *Lancet*, **335**, 265–9

65. Ryde, S.J.S., Bowen-Simpkins, K., Bowen-Simpkins, P., Evans, W.D., Morgan, W.D. and Compston, J.E. (1994). The effects of oestradiol implants on regional and total bone mass: a three-year longitudinal study. *Clin. Endocrinol.*, **40**, 33–6

66. Studd, J.W.W., Savvas, M., Fogelman, I., Garbett, T., Watson, N.R. and Cooper, D. (1990). The relationship between plasma oestradiol and the increase in bone density in postmenopausal women following treatment with subcutaneous hormone implants. *Am. J. Obstet. Gynecol.*, **163**, 1474–9

67. Chambers, T.J., Chow, J.W.M., Lean, J.M. and Tobias, J.H. (1994). The anabolic action of estrogen on bone. In Ziegler, R., Pfeilschifter, J. and Bräutigam, M. (eds.) *Sex Steroids and Bone*, pp. 19–28. (Berlin, Heidelberg, New York: Springer-Verlag)

68. Chapuy, M.-C., Arlot, M.E., Delmas, P.D. and Meunier, P.D. (1994). Effect of cholecalciferol treatment for three years on hip fractures in elderly women. *Br. Med. J.*, **308**, 1081–2

69. Jones, G., Nguyen, T., Sambrook, P., Kelly, P.J. and Eisman, J.A. (1994). Progressive loss of bone from the femoral neck in elderly people: longitudinal findings from the Dubbo osteoporosis epidemiology study. *Br. Med. J.*, **309**, 691–5

70. Nevitt, M.C., Johnell, P., Black, D.M., Ensrud, K., Genant, H.K. and Cummings, S.R. (1994). Bone mineral density predicts non-spine fractures in very elderly women. *Osteoporosis Int.*, **4**, 325–31

71. Compston, J.E. (1994). Hormone replacement therapy for osteo-porosis: clinical and pathophysiological aspects. *Reproductive Medicine Review*, Vol. 3, pp. 209–24

72. Compston, J.E. (1995). Osteoporosis, corticosteroids and inflammatory bowel disease. *Alimentary Pharmacology and Therapeutics*, Vol. 19, pp. 237–50. (Oxford: Blackwell Scientific Publications)

6

Gonadotrophin releasing hormone analogues: the pharmacological model of the menopause

R. W. Shaw

INTRODUCTION

The gonadotrophin releasing hormone (GnRH) agonist analogues have now been established as effective options for a wide variety of benign gynaecological conditions. They are indicated for their specific ability to reduce basal gonadotrophin levels and prevent pulsatile gonadotrophin secretion (in precocious puberty, polycystic ovary syndrome) or to prevent a positive feedback surge of gonadotrophins which finalize follicle maturation and oocyte release (in selective ovulation induction cycles, or in assisted conception treatments). However, their principle facility is the reversible suppression of ovarian function and lowering of circulating oestrogen levels. Conditions that have been treated by this approach include endometriosis, uterine fibroids, dysfunctional uterine bleeding, preparation of the endometrium for transcervical ablation, pre-menstrual syndrome and oestrogen-dependent breast carcinoma. For many of these conditions the requirement is for relatively long-term therapy with GnRH analogues, particularly in conditions such as endometriosis where often a minimum of 6 months suppressive therapy is currently utilized. For most of the above conditions the administration of GnRH agonists is not curative since it has been observed that the clinical effects tend to be reduced or completely negated once ovarian function returns to normal.

Whilst relatively free of any specific side-effects related to the compounds, GnRH agonists induce persistently lowered levels of oestradiol. These cause menopausal vasomotor and psychosomatic symptoms which, although well tolerated by the majority of patients in comparison to symptoms related to the disease the drugs are being administered for, can be problematic. However, there is one serious effect of long-term induced hypo-oestrogenism – altered bone metabolism. Prolonged sustained oestrogen deprivation in premenopausal women from whatever cause, has a significant impact with an accelerated rate of loss of trabecular bone, which appears to be particularly oestrogen sensitive. As a result of these problems, the GnRH agonists' use has to be of the shortest duration necessary for the treatment of the condition and many drug regulatory authorities have limited their use to a period of 6 months. This is likely to change when more data are accrued on longer term administration effects or appropriate regimens have been developed where concomitant administration of other agents prevent the bone loss effects of sustained hypo-oestrogenism.

Administration of GnRH agonists can thus act as a model of the menopause in terms of biochemical and symptomatic changes induced by their lowering of circulating oestrogen.

ADVERSE EFFECTS EXPERIENCED DURING GnRH ANALOGUE THERAPY

In many patients receiving medical therapy for a benign gynaecological condition the adverse effects of the administered drug therapy may be as severe or, in some instances, less desirable or unacceptable than their disease symptoms.

The adverse effects reported during GnRH agonists use result from the hypo-oestrogenaemia induced. The likely character of the adverse effects experienced may be predicted as 'menopausal-like' symptoms. These are particularly hot flushes, vaginal dryness, loss of libido, fatigue and headaches, and tend to increase in their overall frequency with longer duration of use of the agents. The

Table 1 Commonest adverse side effects reported in trials utilizing GnRH analogues

	Goserelin[25] 3.6 mg depot (monthly)	Nafarelin[26] 400 µg/day i.n.	Buserelin[27] 200 µg/day s.c 1200 µg/day i.n.
Number	204	171	116
Percentages of patients with:			
Hot flushes	98	98	71
Vaginal dryness	71	18	29
Decreased libido	66	17	9
Headaches	5	9	23
Weight gain	1	1	1
Breast pain	5	11	n/a
Nausea	5	2	2
Muscle cramps	1	2	2
Acne	37	16	6
Oily skin	25	n/a	n/a
Mood changes (depression/emotional lability)	50	7	10

s.c. = subcutaneously, n/a = not asked, i.n. = intranasally

frequency of a particular side-effect depends upon the relative degree of oestrogen suppression achieved by the various GnRH agonist preparations but more probably on the population studied and the specific questions asked during a trial. The incidence of the two main adverse effects, that of hot flushes and vaginal dryness, can vary between 70 and 95% (hot flushes) and 18 and 71% (vaginal dryness) in the various studies reported.

The incidence of side-effects is reported in a number of randomized trials comparing GnRH analogues, as tabulated in Table 1. Whilst the side-effects appear to be relatively common, perhaps the relative severity of their symptoms is better judged by the proportion of patients who discontinue therapy because of them. In most trials continuation before completion of treatment has been relatively low in those patients randomized to receive GnRH agonists. In one study, the European Goserelin Trial, a significant difference between

Table 2 Methods of measuring bone mass and their accuracy

Technique	Precision (%)	Absorbed dose radiation (mrem)	Site
Single-photon absorptiometry (SPA)	1–3	10–20	Proximal/distal radius
Dual energy photon absorptiometry (DPA)	2–4	5	Spine, hip, total body
Dual energy X-ray absorptiometry (DEXA)	0.5–2	1–3	Spine, hip, total body
Quantitative computerized tomography (QCT)	2–5	100–1000	Spine

the number of drop-outs in patients receiving goserelin 3.6 mg depot every 28 days was 2 out of 204 (1%), compared with those randomized to danazol 600 mg daily, where 10 of 103 patients (9.5%), ceased therapy during the treatment phase. This was a significant difference – $p < 0.05$. Other studies also reported a significant rate of the proportion of the patients discontinuing danazol therapy. This indicates that the hypo-oestrogenic adverse effects induced by GnRH agonists are perhaps better tolerated than the androgenic anabolic effects induced by danazol. This may be an important factor in determining the choice of medical therapy, particularly in patients with recurrent disease who may have been intolerant to previous drug therapy. In many patients, however, the hypo-oestrogenic side-effects are problematic and methods to reduce or completely suppress them, via the use of addback therapy, are being sought.

MECHANISMS OF CHANGES IN BONE MASS

The hypo-oestrogenism induced by GnRH agonists exerts its effect on bone mineral mass through three target tissue sites.

(1) Parathyroid action

Oestrogen stimulates calcitonin secretion and antagonizes the peripheral action of parathyroid hormone. Decreased oestrogen levels will therefore reduce parathyroid secretion of calcitonin, leading to decreased total body calcium allowing unrestrained parathyroid hormone activity and an increase in bone resorption.

(2) Action within bone

Oestrogen-like receptors are present in osteoblasts or osteoblast-like cells[1]. Lowered circulatory oestrogen levels reduce oestrogen receptor activity, resulting in decreased mineral deposition and reduced bone formation. Transforming growth factor beta (TGF beta) and insulin-like factor I (IGF I) both stimulate bone formation and are thought to be influenced by oestrogen[2]. In addition, they inhibit prostaglandin E_2 and interleukin which are known to stimulate bone resorption. In situations of reduced oestrogen circulating levels (such as those induced by GnRH agonists) decreased bone formation and increased bone resorption occur simultaneously.

(3) Intestinal absorption with calcium

Decreased oestrogen levels lead to decreased conversion of vitamin D to 1,25-dihydroxyvitamin D (a known oestrogen-dependent process). The result is poorer intestinal absorption of calcium, reduced levels of 1,25-dihydroxyvitamin D and such changes have been reported during continued administration of GnRH agonists[3].

CHANGES IN BONE BIOCHEMISTRY

The earliest detectable changes in bone biochemistry following commencement of GnRH agonist therapy are those of raised urinary calcium:creatinine and hydroxyproline:creatinine ratios[4,5]. These changes reflect an increase in bone resorption following the withdrawal of the protective effects of normal circulating levels of oestrogen and their protective effect on the skeleton. In a normal bone remodelling cycle, there is coupling between resorption and new bone formation. Thus after an increase in resorption there would be evidence of an increase in parameters reflecting bone formation. Currently the commonest biochemical measurements used to assess bone formation are the measurement of serum alkaline phosphatase and serum osteocalcin. Both alkaline phosphatase and osteocalcin are seen to rise significantly after 6 months treatment with GnRH agonist[3,6]. Clearly if only changes occurred which reflected increased bone absorption or, alternatively, those parameters reflecting bone formation, then major changes in bone structure could be predicted. However, if both parameters of resorption and formation are altered simultaneously it is more difficult to predict from biochemical measurements what precisely is happening within the bone structure. For these reasons it is necessary to rely upon physical measurements of bone mineral concentration and bone mineral density to reflect changes of the *status quo* within bone.

BONE MINERAL DENSITY MEASUREMENTS

There are a number of methods currently available for measuring bone mass which vary in accuracy and precision with differences in absorbed doses of radiation (Table 2). Bone mass is calculated on the basis of tissue absorption of photons derived from an X-ray tube of radionucleotides. The method of bone mineral density (BMD) measurement and the specific bone site studied will give some variability of results. However, there are now abundant data from both double-blind and open non-randomized studies indicating significant measurable loss in trabecular bone as early as 3 months after commencement of GnRH agonist therapy in patients treated for endometriosis[7]. Most studies that have used dual photon absorbtiometry (DPA) or dual energy X-ray absorbtiometry (DEXA) have indicated a mean reduction of 5–6% reduction in BMD within the predominantly trabecular bone of the lumbar spine (L2–L4) and a loss of 3–4% of the mixed trabecular and cortical bone in Ward's triangle (femoral neck). Studies of predominantly cortical bone in the femoral shaft show losses of 1.7–1.8% which, because of the sensitivity of the detection methods, is not significantly different from baseline control groups (see Table 2).

Follow-up studies show a return towards baseline BMD with time in most patients, once GnRH agonist therapy has stopped and ovarian function has recommenced with return of normal circulating premenopausal oestrogen levels. There can, however, be a time lag of up to 12 months in many individuals before BMDs approach their pretreatment baseline values. BMD alters with age and the fact that there is a gradual loss of between 0.5 and 1% per annum following the years of peak bone mass attainment (approximately age 35–40 years), some individuals may never return to apparent baseline BMD. This may merely reflect the expected age-related change reduction. The association between loss of ovarian function and osteoporosis is beyond dispute[8,9]. Additionally, Cann and co-workers[10] demonstrated a slight deviation in cortical bone and up to a 20% decrease in spinal trabecular bone (measured by QCT) in amenorrhoeic women with hypothalamic or hyperprolactinaemia amenorrhoea or premature ovarian failure. These studies indicate that it is not only menopausal women who are at risk of a reduction in bone mineral content and that the changes observed following the hypo-oestrogenic state induced by GnRH agonists are not unique and are similar to those observed in premenopausal women in whom a state of hypo-oestrogenism occurs, be it physiological or pharmacologically induced.

Increase in bone mineral, on the other hand, has been demonstrated when appropriately dosed oestrogen replacement treatment has been commenced within a few years of the natural or surgically induced menopause, achieving restoration of some or all of that lost[11,12]. We would thus expect regain of bone mineral content to occur following cessation of GnRH A therapy and resumption of normal ovarian function.

The degree of bone loss seen in patients treated with GnRH agonist therapy for periods of 6 months has no immediate clinical or likely long-term effects within bone and these patients remain asymptomatic. However, such reductions in BMD without complete replacement, in women with recurrent disease conditions who may inevitably require repeat courses of treatment with GnRH agonists will have a cumulative effect and ultimately a negative impact on peak bone mass and potential long-term implications for fracture risk. Thus, if GnRH A were used in the longer term its effect on bone mass would be of concern. West and colleagues[13] assessed women after 12 months of GnRH agonist therapy and noted an 8% spinal bone loss. For these reasons strategies to avoid or prevent such bone losses are being developed. The concept of addback therapy aims to counteract the hypo-oestrogenic side-effects, including bone loss, without stimulating the condition for which the GnRH agonist had originally been given and thus introduces the possibility of extended treatment courses. Benign gynaecological conditions for which long-term treatment would potentially be utilized include endometriosis, dysfunctional uterine bleeding and fibroids, since following short-term treatment courses there is a tendency for the disease to recur with increase in time, and return of ovarian function. When using GnRH agonists it is important to select patients with a low risk of osteoporosis. Increased risk is associated with a family history of the condition, smoking and high alcohol consumption, caucasian or oriental origin, low dietary calcium intake (less than 800 mg/day) and low body mass index.

An alternative approach is a multi-agent therapy to neutralize the hypo-oestrogenic-induced side-effects as well as the bone-depleting side-effects of GnRH agonists. A variety of agents have been investigated as potential addback therapies. These include progestogens or oestrogens alone, oestrogen/progestogen (HRT) preparations, tibolone, etidronate, calcitonin or parathyroid hormone. These regimens produce different results in terms of relieving hypo-oestrogenic side-effects with sodium etidronate, calcium carbonate, calcitonin, parathormone, potentially providing bone protection but having no effect on hypo-oestrogenic symptoms. For these reasons other addback regimens have been further investigated, including various progestogens, oestrogen/progestogen combinations and tibolone.

PROGESTOGENS

Progestogens seem an ideal addback regimen as when administered alone, in the absence of oestrogen, they have been shown to inhibit bone loss and alleviate menopausal symptoms[14,15]. The choice would also seem logical since all of the conditions for which GnRH agonists long-term are being administered are oestrogen-dependent (endometriosis, uterine fibroids). The first randomized prospective trial to assess GnRH agonists alone – or in combination with a progestogenic agent – was in women with symptomatic endometriosis[16]. These women were given leuprolide depot monthly with placebo or depot plus 5 mg norethisterone daily for 4 weeks increased to 10 mg daily for a further 20 weeks. Patients receiving addback therapy had significantly less hot flushes and reduced vaginal symptoms than the analogue alone group and the percentage decrease in BMD in the analogue alone group was $5.6 \pm 0.7\%$ versus $2.7 \pm 0.7\%$ in the addback group as assessed by DEXA in the lumbar spine. There was a significant reduction in HDL and an increase in LDL/HDL ratio in the norethisterone addback group. Both regimens successfully eliminated visible endometriotic implants and relieved the symptoms attributable to endometriosis.

Medroxyprogesterone acetate (MPA) at a dose of 15 mg a day versus placebo has also been evaluated in patients with fibroids treated with goserelin 3.6 mg depot[13]. MPA or placebo were started 12 weeks after commencement with goserelin treatment. Commencement immediately with addback therapy failed to allow any reduction in fibroid size, thus the above strategy was necessary. The addition of MPA had no detrimental effect, compared to placebo, on maintenance of fibroid shrinkage but did relieve hypo-oestrogen effects significantly when compared with placebo. However, this combination failed to protect bone loss since the MPA group had a decrease of 7% in spinal BMD (compared to 7.7% in the placebo group).

OESTROGEN AND PROGESTOGEN COMBINATIONS

Clearly the administration of oestrogen is proven to control hypo-oestrogenic symptoms as well as, if given in appropriate doses, prevent bone loss. However, administration of unopposed oestrogens, even at relatively small doses, could lead to prevention or reduction of GnRH agonists effect on the disease processes for which they had been administered. This would be of particular concern in endometriosis and uterine fibroids.

In one study[17], patients with uterine fibroids were randomized to receive leuprolide depot alone for 12 weeks then randomized to receive oestropipate 0.7 mg daily with 0.7 mg norethisterone on days 1–14 of each month or norethisterone 10 mg daily. In both groups on initial GnRH agonist alone treatment for 3 months there was a 64% decrease in mean uterine volume. The administration of oestrogen and progesterone did not result in regrowth of the fibroids during continuation of the study over a further 9 months of treatment whereas in the progestogen alone group there was a tendency for regrowth of the fibroid over the ensuing 40 weeks. Significant bone loss in the lumbar spine occurred during the first 3 months, of between 2.7 to 3.3% with a further loss of 2% between weeks 12 and 52 in the oestrogen/progesterone group, but a 0.8% gain in the progesterone alone group. Neither of these changes were significantly different from the 3-month GnRH-alone time assessment. Lipoprotein changes in terms of lowering of HDL occurred in the progesterone alone group compared with the oestrogen/progesterone group and there were also more unscheduled bleeding episodes in the progesterone alone group than the oestrogen/progesterone group[17].

Maheux and Lemay[18] also studied patients with uterine fibroids and treated them with goserelin depot alone for 3 months followed then by conjugated oestrogen 0.3 mg and MGA 5 mg daily. Initial reduction in fibroid volume was just under 50% which was maintained when addback therapy was commenced. There was satisfactory control of hypo-oestrogenic symptoms with this particular combination but bone changes in the lumbar spine were not completely prevented since over 6 months a 6.7% reduction in BMD (as assessed by DEXA) of the lumbar spine occurred.

With endometriosis there was perhaps more concern about the use of any form of oestrogenic addback therapy. However, Howell and co-workers[19] studied 50 patients in an open randomized controlled trial of patients receiving goserelin 3.6 mg monthly for 6 months or goserelin plus transdermal oestradiol 25 mg patch twice weekly and MPA 5 μg daily. In this study, 6 months after commencement of therapy lumbar spine density (as assessed by DEXA) had decreased significantly in both groups but in the group receiving addback treatment the BMD loss was reduced at –2.07% compared with –4.27% in the goserelin alone group. There was control of hypo-oestrogenic symptoms in the addback group and no impairment of impact on the reductions in AFS scores by the use of this low dose addback regimen.

It is true to say that further studies utilizing oestrogen/progestogen combinations in endometriosis utilizing higher levels of oestrogen, enough to completely prevent bone loss, have not as yet been published. However, in one study oestradiol valerate 2 mg together with norethisterone 1 mg daily were given for 6 months, in conjunction with goserelin depot, compared with goserelin depot plus placebo. The results demonstrated excellent control of menopausal symptoms in the addback group with no impaired impact on the endometriosis as assessed at laparoscopy, but the researcher had not reported bone changes in this particular study[20].

The best regimen for oestrogen/progestogen replacement addback treatment in endometriosis is still therefore to be determined.

Tibolone

Tibolone is a synthetic steroid with weak progestogenic, androgenic and oestrogenic properties and has been used as a single agent HRT preparation in post-menopausal women where it has been shown to relieve menopausal symptoms and prevent bone loss yet not stimulate the endometrium[21,22]. We have reported[23] a study utilizing tibolone as addback therapy in 33 patients predominantly with endometriosis who were randomized to receive the depot analogue triptorelin 3.75 mg monthly with placebo daily or triptorelin plus

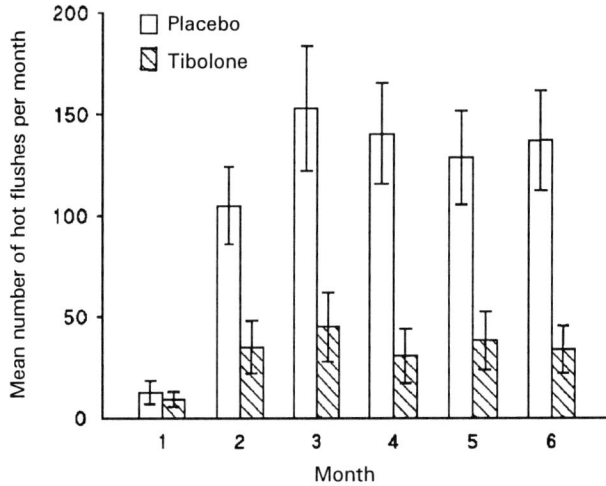

Figure 1 Mean number of flushes per month in patients receiving triptorelin and placebo or triptorelin and addback therapy with tibolone 2.5 mg daily

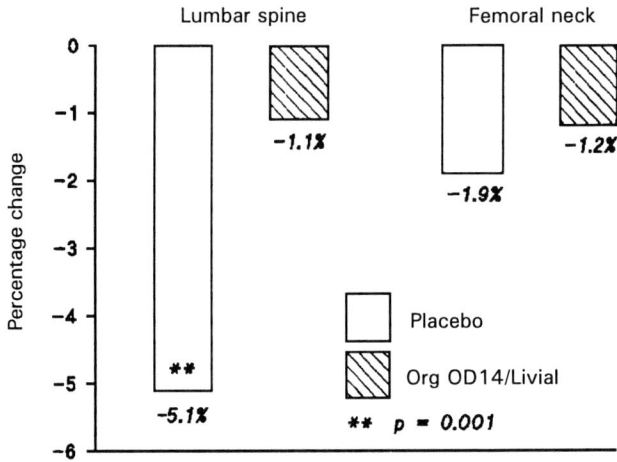

Figure 2 Bone Mineral Density changes following 6 months treatment with triptorelin and placebo or triptorelin and addback therapy of tibolone 2.5 mg daily

tibolone 2.5 mg daily for a total of 24 weeks. The patients receiving tibolone as addback therapy had significantly less hot flushes and indeed 50% of patients had no hot flushes whatsoever (Figure 1). Both the groups showed comparable and significant reductions in AFS and ADI endometriosis scores. With regard to bone loss the placebo treated group lost 5.1% of BMD in the lumbar vertebrae (Figure 2) (as assessed by DEXA) compared with 1.1% in the tibolone addback group. At the femoral neck the bone loss was greater in the placebo group but this was not significantly different from the addback treated group. The effect of tibolone on lipids was not reported in this study but previous authors had reported a decrease in total cholesterol-triglyceride and in the HDL-cholesterol component of lipoproteins[24].

Tibolone therefore appears to have great potential as an effective therapy as it appears to act on the bone in a way comparable to oestrogen, is more potent than progestogens, and yet does not have the stimulatory effects of oestrogen on the endometrium or on endometriosis. Likewise, in the comparative trial reported above[24] a number of patients underwent bone biopsies. The administration of tibolone prevented the significant changes, as seen by morphometry, compared with the group treated with GnRH analogue alone. These findings have been reported and discussed in Chapter 5 by Dr Compston.

CONCLUSIONS

Without doubt GnRH analogue therapies are effective in a number of benign gynaecological conditions. Continued use results in significant reduction of circulating oestrogen levels and induces hypo-oestrogenic side-effects. The side-effects, whilst well tolerated by the majority of patients, can be troublesome and means to relieve them should be sought. A significant effect of the hypo-oestrogenism is a reduction in bone mineral density which should be counteracted by use of addback treatment when prolonged (more than 6 months) or repeated treatment cycles of GnRH analogues are contemplated. The ideal addback regimen for the various conditions for which GnRH analogues are utilized have not been determined in many instances at this point in time.

REFERENCES

1. Eriksen, E.F., Colvard, D.S., Berg, N.J., Graham, M.L., Mann, K.G., Spelsburg, T.C. and Riggs, B.L. (1988). Evidence of oestrogen receptors in normal human osteoblast-like cells. *Science*, **241**, 81–4
2. Ernst, M., Schmid, C., Frankenfoldt, C. and Froesch, E.R. (1988). Estradiol stimulation of osteoblast proliferation *in vitro*. Mediator roles for TGF beta PGF2 IGF1.(Abstr) *Calcif. Tiss. Res.*, **42**, (Suppl. 117)
3. Scharla, H.S., Minne, H.W., Waibel-Treber, S., Schaible, A., Lempert, U.G., Wüster, C., Leyendecker, G. and Ziegler, R. (1990). Bone mass reduction after oestrogen deprivate by long acting gonadotropin-releasing hormone agonists and its relation to pretreatment concentrations of 1,25-dihydroxyvitamin D3. *J. Clin. Endocrinol. Metab.*, **70**, 1055–61
4. Bergquist, C. (1990). Effects of nafarelin versus danazol on lipids and calcium metabolism. *Am. J. Obstet. Gynecol.*, **162**, 589–91
5. Gudmundsson, J.A., Lyunghall, S., Bergquist, C., Wide, L. and Nillius, S.J. (1987). Increased bone turnover during gonadotropin-releasing hormone super-agonist-induced ovulation inhibition. *J. Clin. Endocrinol. Metab.*, **65**, 159–63
6. Ylikorkala, O., Nilsson, C.G., Hirvonen, E. and Viinikka, L. (1990). Evidence of similar increases in bone turnover during nafarelin and danazol use in women with endometriosis. *Gynecol. Endocrinol.*, **4**, 251–60
7. Dawood, M.Y. (1994). Hormonal therapies for endometriosis: implications for bone metabolism. *Acta Obstet. Gynecol. Scand.*, **159** (Suppl. 2–34)
8. Christiensen, M.S., McNair, P., Hagen, C., Stocklund, K., Transbol, I. (1980). Prevention of early postmenopausal bone loss: controlled two-year study in 315 normal females. *Eur. J. Clin. Invest.*, **10**, 273–279
9. Al Azzawi, F., Hart, D.M., Lindsay, R. (1987). Long term effect of oestrogen replacement therapy on bone mass as measured by dual photon absorptiometry. *Br. Med. J.*, **294**, 1261–2
10. Cann, C.E., Henzl, M., Burry, K. *et al.* (1987). Reversible bone loss is produced by the GnRH agonist Nafarelin. In Cohn, D.V., Martin, T.J., Meunier, L. (eds.) *Calcium Regulations and Bone Metabolism: Basic*

     and Clinical Aspects, pp. 123–7. (Amsterdam: Elsevier Science Publications)

11.   Christiansen, C., Christiansen, M.S. and Transbol, I. (1981). Bone mass in menopausal women after withdrawal of oestrogen/gestagen replacement therapy. *Lancet*, **1**, 459–61

12.   Lindsay, R., Hart, D.M., Forrest, C.A. and Baird, C. (1980). Prevention of osteoporosis in oophorectomised women. *Lancet*, **2**, 1151–4

13.   West, C.P., Lumsden, M.A., Lawson, S., Williamson, J. and Baird, D.T. (1987). Shrinkage of uterine fibroids during therapy with goserelin ('Zoladex'): a luteinizing hormone-releasing hormone agonist administered as a monthly subcutaneous depot. *Fertil. Steril.*, **48**, 45–51

14.   Paterson, M.E.L. (1982). A randomised double-blinded cross-over trial into the effects of norethisterone on climacteric symptoms and biochemical profiles. *Br. J. Obstet. Gynaecol.*, **89**, 464–72

15.   Abdalla, H.I., Hart, D.M., Lindsay, R., Leggate, I. and Hooke, A. (1985). Prevention of bone mineral loss in postmenopausal women by norethisterone. *Obstet. Gynecol.*, **66**, 789–92

16.   Surrey, E.S. and Judd, H.L. (1992). Reduction of vasomotor symptoms and bone mineral density loss with combined norethindrone and long-acting gonadotrophin-releasing hormone agonist therapy of symptomatic endometriosis: a prospective randomised trial. *J. Clin. Endocrinol. Metab.*, **75**, 558–53

17.   Friedman, A.J., Daly, E., Juneau-Norcross, M., Gleason, R., Rein, M.S. and LeBoff, M. (1994). Long-term medical therapy for leiomyomata uteri: a prospective, randomized study of leuprolide acetate depot plus either oestrogen-progestin or progestin "Add-Back" for two years. *Hum. Reprod.*, **9**, 1618–25

18.   Maheux, R. and Lemay, A. (1992). Treatment of peri-menopausal women: potential long-term therapy with a depot GnRH agonist combined with hormonal replacement therapy. *Br. J. Obstet. Gynaecol.*, **99** (Suppl. 13–17)

19.   Edmonds, D.K. and Howell, R. (1994). Can hormone replacement therapy be used during medical therapy of endometriosis? *Br. J. Obstet. Gynaecol.*, **101** (Suppl. 10), 24–6

20.   Kiilholma, P., Tuimala, R., Kivinen, S., Korhonen, M. and Hagman, E. (1996). Comparison of the GnRH-A goserelin acetate alone vs goserelin combined with estrogen-progestogen addback therapy in the treatment of endometriosis. *Fertil. Steril.*, in press

21.   Benedek-Jaszman L.J. (1987). Long term placebo-controlled efficacy and safety study of ORG OD14 in climacteric women. *Maturitas*, (Suppl. 1, 25–33)

22. Punnonen, R., Liukko, P., Corte-Prieto, J., Eydam, F., Mitojevic, S., Trevoux, R., Chryssikopoulos, E., Franchi, F., Luisi, M. and Kicovic, P.M. (1984). Multicentre study of effects of ORG14 on endometrium vaginal cytology and cervical mucus in post-menopausal and oophorectomized women. *Maturitas*, **5**, 281–6

23. Lindsay, P.C., Shaw, R.W., Coelingh Bennink, H.J. and Kicovic, P. (1996). The effect of addback treatment with tibolone (Livial) on patients treated with the gonadotropin releasing hormone agonist triptorelin (Decapeptyl). *Fertil. Steril.*, **65**, 342–48

24. Farish, E., Barnes, J.F., Rolton, H.A., Spowart, K., Fletcher, D.C. and Hart, D.M. (1994). Effect of tibolone on lipoprotein (a) and HDL subfractions. *Maturitas*, **20**, 215–9

25. Shaw, R.W. (1992). An open randomised comparative study of the effect of goserelin and danazol in the treatment of endometriosis. *Fertil Steril.*, **58**, 265–72

26. The Nafarelin European Endometriosis Group. (1992). A large scale danazol controlled trial of efficacy and safety with one year follow-up. *Fertil. Steril.*, **57**, 514–22

27. Protocol 310 Study Group. (1990). A comparison of the efficacy and safety of buserelin vs. danazol in the treatment of endometriosis. In Chanda, D.R. and Buttram, V.C. Jr (eds.) *Current Concepts in Endometriosis*, pp. 253–67. (New York: Alan R. Liss)

7

Osteoporosis: screening and prevention in younger women

D.W. Purdie

INTRODUCTION

The treatment of established osteoporosis is not easy. Once substantial amounts of bone tissue have been lost from key areas of spine, femoral neck and distal radius it is extremely difficult to make good the deficits. Hence the aim of health commissioners in developed countries where osteoporosis is prevalent should be to develop public health and specialist services whereby the *prevention* of osteoporosis becomes the central goal. To this end we shall consider some of the measures which may be deployed in younger women, before the age of natural menopause, in order to conserve bone mass.

Osteoporosis has recently been redefined qualitatively and also quantitatively in terms of bone mineral density (BMD). The World Health Organization endorsed in 1994 the proposal of a Consensus Development Conference that definition of osteoporosis should be: *a disease characterized by low bone mass and microarchitectural deterioration of bone tissue, leading to enhanced fragility and a consequent increase in fracture risk*[1]. In hard numbers, WHO has now also proposed that the disease be deemed present when BMD has fallen below 2.5 standard deviations (SDs) below the mean value for young healthy persons in that population. Similarly, the intermediate condition of osteopenia is deemed present when the BMD value

Table 1 Bone mineral density (BMD) changes at generalized life stages

Life stage	*Bone mineral density*
Fetal life (40 weeks)	gain
Childhood and puberty (<15 years)	gain
Early adulthood (15–25 years)	gain
Maturity (25–50 years)	steady state
Postmenopause (>50 years)	loss

Maintenance of the premenopausal steady state is contingent on normal ovarian function

falls between 1.0 and 2.5 SD below the young normal mean. The number of SD above or below the mean is conveniently referred to as a 'T' score[2]. Thus osteoporosis is present when $T > -2.5$. The central medical goal, therefore, is to maintain BMD as close as possible to that of young healthy persons in whom the risk of fracture is minimal.

Bone strength is highly correlated with BMD and is built up during childhood and adolescence to a peak bone mass which is achieved, though at different times for different bones, usually during the third decade[3] (Table 1).

INTRAUTERINE LIFE

We know that bone is laid down during fetal life and that the fetal skeleton is fuelled with calcium largely between 28 weeks and term[4]. The newborn infant continues to accrete calcium in the skeleton and this process proceeds unabated till puberty. In girls the advent of cyclic ovarian activity introduces oestrogen into the system and this steroid plays a central role in bone physiology henceforward.

It is worth noting at this point that bone, whatever the age of an individual, is a constantly active tissue. In health, bone is formed and removed in a balanced manner which encompasses sites of removal/formation known as bone remodelling units (BRU). In adult humans some 500 000 of these microscopic sites are in action at any one time. The basic timescale for the operation of a BRU is shown in Table 2.

Table 2 The sequence of events in the bone remodelling cycle at a bone remodelling unit

Activity	Cell	Duration (weeks)
Resorption	Osteoclast	2–3
Resting phase	—	2–3
Formation	Osteoblast	6–7

It is generally agreed that genetic factors contribute significantly to peak bone mass and this has been strongly supported by mother-daughter examinations[5] and twin studies[6]. However, environmental influences also play a part in modulating peak bone mass and among these the principal determinants are calcium intake and physical exercise. The first opportunity for health professionals to influence the development of a healthy skeleton is therefore to advocate to parents, schoolteachers and public health officials, on appropriate dietary calcium intake[7] and physical exercise[8]. The principal non-environmental factor which may affect bone behaviour in women is the menstrual cycle, or rather the circulating level of oestradiol. Any condition which results in a fall in plasma oestrogen to levels seen in postmenopausal women (<150 pmol/l) will result in loss of bone.

OVARIAN DYSGENESIS

Primary amenorrhoea as seen most frequently in cases of Turner's syndrome has been found to be associated with extremely low values of BMD. Indeed in a comparative survey Davies and colleagues[9] reported that the reduction in bone mass was greatest in women who were amenorrhoeic due to ovarian dysgenesis. These women should be offered oestrogen replacement either with the combined oral-contraceptive pill or with hormone replacement therapy (HRT) preparations. However, it remains to be seen if the exhibition of oestrogen is associated with a prolonged and significant bone gain.

ANOREXIA NERVOSA

Anorexia nervosa and related conditions have a prevalence of up to 4% in young women[10]. Kaplan and co-workers[11] reported a high prevalence of severe osteopenia in anorexic women and the bone loss may be sufficient to provoke fracture after minimal or moderate trauma. In a prospective study, Klibanski and colleagues[12] noted that bone density at the spine was, as expected, lower in anorexics than controls. However, they were not able to demonstrate that oestrogen can reverse, let alone arrest, bone loss in such patients. Interestingly, those subjects whose anorexia nervosa remitted spontaneously with a return to menstruation, did manifest a gain in bone density. This suggests the intriguing possibility that endocrine factors other than oestrogen and progesterone may operate during the menstrual cycle to protect bone. Further studies are required in this area.

HYPERPROLACTINAEMIA

Another cause of secondary hypoestrogenaemia which will come within the practice of the gynaecologist is hyperprolactinaemia. As is usual when oestrogen deficiency is the provoking cause, bone loss is most severe at trabecular bone sites, particularly the spine. Such losses have been reported to be as high as 25% when compared to healthy controls[13]. The effect is believed to be due to the suppressive action of prolactin upon gonadotrophic hormone production and hence ovarian function rather than to an intrinsic action of prolactin itself. In a prospective study of 43 hyperprolactir.aemic women Schlechte and colleagues[14] found that the hyperprolactinaemic group did indeed have a significantly lower spinal BMD than controls but that the value was in steady state. They also observed that BMD did not normalize when treatment with trans-sphenoidal surgery or with bromocriptine resulted in a resumption of gonadal function. There thus appears to be a significant difference between the bone loss which attends natural menopause and that which is consequent on hyperprolactinaemia. It has been reported that the bone loss in such women occurs soon after the onset of hyperprolactinaemia and is present by 2 years from diagnosis[15]. The above data have clinical

104

relevance in that they suggest that osteopenia need not be a clamant indication for treatment in, for example, hyperprolactinaemic women without macroprolactinomas who are well and do not desire fertility. Recently, however, Biller and co-workers[16] have reported that restoration of menses in treated patients improved trabecular bone density in just over half the patients studied.

ATHLETES

Another group of young women who have come in for much attention in recent years are school and college athletes. Marcus and colleagues[17] observed that oligomenorrhoeic athletes, whose menstrual dysfunction was due to a training-induced reduction in fat mass, have a lower BMD than eumenorrhoeic controls. The relationship between BMD and oligomenorrhoea was further explored by Lloyd and associates[18] who showed that the decrement in bone density was strongly correlated with the precise number of menses which had been missed. Using quantitative computed tomography (QCT) Wolman and co-workers[19] showed that extensive exercise can only partially compensate for bone loss sustained by amenorrhoeic athletes from various disciplines studied at the British Olympic Medical Centre. Not surprisingly BMD reduction in athletes may lead to stress fractures. In a study of South African athletes who had sustained such fractures it was found that patients were more likely than controls to have menstrual dysfunction and related low bone density[20].

The therapeutic use of gonadotrophin releasing hormone (GnRH) agonists for 6 months, usually in the management of endometriosis is associated with profound hypoestrogenaemia and has been shown to result in a rapid loss of bone which may be reversible after terminating treatment[21]. However, Shaw[22] has cautioned that prolonged use of GnRH analogues will require the development and successful trial of 'add-back' oestrogen replacement regimens.

These conditions and circumstances provide a vivid illustration of the primacy of oestrogen in the protection of the female skeleton. Young athletes, for example, are clinically well, have diets replete in calcium and exercise maximally, yet they lose bone, perhaps to an irreversible degree if their hypothalamic-ovarian function is sufficiently compromised to depress ambient plasma oestradiol below the bone protection threshold.

Thus there is cause for concern in all circumstances in which menstrual function is lost or disrupted and where plasma oestrogen levels are below the normal premenopausal range. General practitioners and gynaecologists should be alert to the need for full investigation of primary or secondary amenorrhoea and for the provision of replacement oestrogen for bone protection where indicated.

PREGNANCY AND LACTATION

There is a considerable literature relating to the reproductive cycle and bone mineral density. Given that pregnancy and lactation exert substantial effects on calcium homeostasis the central aim has been to enquire if the skeleton exits the reproductive cycle with significant change in the key area of BMD. With regard to pregnancy Purdie and colleagues[23] showed that although bone mass was mobilized in early gestation to provide available calcium for both maternal and fetal needs, this process was reversed at term with losses being made good. With regard to lactation, Sowers and co-workers[24] examined the effect of breast feeding for over 5 months, with BMD being assessed prospectively by dual-energy X-ray absorptiometry. These workers observed, in a well conducted study, that a breast-feeding woman lost bone both at spine (5.1%) and femoral neck (4.8%) over 6 months. They further noted that these losses were cancelled out by postlactational bone recovery, and that BMD was back to baseline levels at 12 months after weaning. Thus it would seem that the reproductive cycle is broadly neutral in respect of the skeleton and the above perinatal studies are indeed in accord with the observation that osteoporosis in older women is not more frequent among higher parity groups.

BONE SCREENING

We now move on to perhaps the most contentious and exciting area of development, namely the debate on the applicability of bone

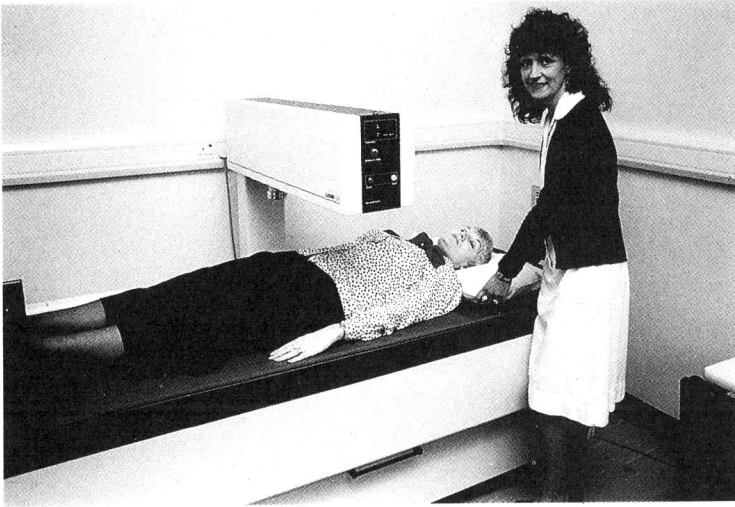

Figure 1 Dual-energy X-ray absorptiometer. The systems installed at Princess Royal Hospital give a precision of approximately 0.8% in spinal bone mineral density measurement

densitometry to the purpose of picking out those individuals destined to develop osteoporosis later. This debate has been triggered by the general agreement that osteoporosis is worthy of prevention, that dual-energy X-ray absorptiometry (DEXA) is a precise and accurate test (Figure 1) and that HRT, if taken in adequate dosage and for long enough, will result in BMD conservation. However, we are still a long way from advocating screening of women as they approach menopause. This is for two principal reasons. First, it has yet to be shown by prospective trial that densitometric testing and selective treatment is associated with a significant reduction in the key clinical end points of spinal and femoral neck fracture. Second, despite recent improvements in delivery systems, compliance with HRT regimens remains poor and is likely to remain so until efficacious amenorrhoeic regimens are available and tested. Furthermore, high compliance will require greater reassurance than that currently available on the safety of combined HRT regimens particularly with respect to the risk of breast cancer.

Nevertheless, certain Health Authorities have been persuaded to fund the performance of bone densitometry on certain groups of the population. The indications for densitometric examination approved by the Public Health and Commissioning Group of East Riding Health in Yorkshire, England, are broadly in line with those advocated by the National Osteoporosis Foundation in the US and the National Osteoporosis Society in the UK.

Oestrogen-deficient women who would wish to be treated or to continue treatment if found to be osteopenic

There are substantial numbers of women who are undecided about HRT at the time of natural or premature menopause and who find decision making difficult when based solely on current symptoms and a family history of, say, osteoporosis or coronary artery disease. These women are offered densitometry on the premise that osteopenia (BMD of 1–2.5 SD below young normal mean) confers a higher lifetime risk of fracture[25]. This may be reduced, up to age 75 years, by the use of at least 7 years of an osteoprotective HRT regimen[26]. At present, HRT prescription in the UK is usually for a period of approximately 18 months and may involve a dose of oestrogen such as the 25 µg patch or 1 mg oestradiol orally which is not osteoprotective. Knowledge of enhanced fracture risk may thus allow the prescribing doctor, usually the general practitioner, to deploy a bone-sparing regimen for an adequate duration, that is, for at least 5 years. For reference, the daily minima of oestrogen required for skeletal protection are: 2 mg oestradiol orally, 0.625 mg of conjugated equine oestrogen orally, 50 µg oestradiol transdermally and 50 mg oestradiol by implant, at 6-monthly intervals.

Patients suspected to be osteoporotic from radiological findings

Standard radiology is a notoriously imprecise method of diagnosing early osteoporosis, yet it has an important part to play in case recognition if only because of its frequency of employment and because when the bones appear radiologically translucent on standard film, it is highly likely that a significant degree of bone loss has occurred. Radiologists generally comment on radiolucency when they observe

Table 3 Medical conditions associated with osteoporosis (incomplete list)

Cushing's syndrome
Thyrotoxicosis
Hyperparathyroidism
Rheumatoid arthritis
Malabsorption syndromes
Postgastrectomy syndrome
Chronic anticonvulsant therapy
Diabetes mellitus

Certain of the above conditions are discussed in the text

it especially when the possibility of osteoporosis has been suggested in the *clinical details* section of the request. This practice should be encouraged locally.

Patients who have a medical condition predisposing to osteoporosis such as thyroid disease, anorexia nervosa, malabsorption syndromes and other rarer causes of osteoporosis

Those medical conditions which adversely affect BMD should be known to practitioners involved in osteoporosis management and prevention. (Table 3). Such conditions include hyperthyroidism, where the mechanism is believed to involve T_4-stimulated activation of osteoclast activity, perhaps mediated by interleukins[27]. More commonly patients presenting with hypothyroidism, treated or untreated, should receive a BMD scan since the hypothyroid state often represents the endstage of a pre-existing hyperthyroidism during which significant bone loss may have occurred. Patients who have undergone thyroidectomy have low plasma calcitonin levels and may develop osteopenia[28].

In type I diabetes mellitus several studies have shown a reduction in cortical bone which would tend to have its greatest impact at the femoral neck where the proportion of cortical to trabecular bone is higher. The mechanism for the bone loss in insulin-dependent diabetes is unclear[29] but may involve renal loss of calcium[30]. Interestingly, individuals suffering from type II, maturity onset diabetes, who are often overweight, do not share the osteopenia of insulin-dependent diabetes. Type II diabetes has been reported to be associated with enhanced bone mass[31] perhaps due to enhanced peripheral conversion of androstenedione to oestrone in adipose tissue[32]. Also in a purely mechanical way, obese persons are better protected from the trauma of falls.

In rheumatoid arthritis a local osteoporosis in proximity to acutely inflamed joints has long been recognized[33]. However, it is now a matter of considerable debate as to whether there is generalized osteopenia of the skeleton in rheumatoid arthritis which is not just attributable to steroid treatment or enforced immobility.

PATIENTS RECEIVING, OR ABOUT TO RECEIVE STEROID THERAPY IN A REGIMEN LIKELY TO IMPAIR BONE METABOLIC FUNCTION

An association between corticosteroid treatment and osteoporosis has long been recognized. The glucocorticoids both inhibit osteoblast function and reduce absorption of calcium from the gut by inhibition of 1,25 dihydroxyvitamin D activity in the intestinal mucosa[34]. The net result is an excess of bone resorption over formation and, ultimately, an excess of fractures[35]. The critical dose at which such effects are seen clinically seems to be about 7.5 mg prednisolone or equivalent daily. Thus it is prudent to measure BMD in patients embarking on such therapy so that bone loss may be monitored and appropriate modification of treatment applied as necessary.

PATIENTS SUSTAINING A PREMATURE MENOPAUSE OR UNDERGOING HYSTERECTOMY WITH OOPHORECTOMY BELOW AGE 45

Some patients sustaining a premature menopause may welcome the absence of the cycle and regard its termination as a release. However, given our current knowledge of the protective effect of oestrogen on the skeleton and cardiovascular system, it is sensible that such patients should be offered HRT unless a contraindication exists.

Bone loss after menopause is rapid for the first 5 years, especially in the trabecular bone of the spine[36]. Thus patients should be encouraged to report premature menopause to their primary care physicians so that a discussion may ensue regarding the use of oestrogen for bone and blood vessel protection. Bilateral oophorectomy results in obligatory and immediate menopause but the position is more complex in respect of the more common procedure of simply hysterectomy. At the present time it is not at all clear why and when a proportion of postoperative patients sustain ovarian failure but this is sufficient to produce an effect on spinal bone mass[37]. Thus patients undergoing simple hysterectomy before the mid-fifth decade should be advised of the symptoms of menopause and urged to report their development. Densitometry in such patients will provide a baseline assessment of fracture risk and allow the appropriate institution and monitoring of antiresorptive therapy.

PATIENTS EXHIBITING STRONG FAMILY HISTORY OF OSTEOPOROSIS

Unusually this comes in the form of a statement by the patient that her mother, or aunts, have exhibited height loss, kyphosis, or repeated fracture. There is a strong hereditary element in BMD[38] and hence younger patients may observe at first hand the effect of the disease in a first degree relative. In such circumstances it is prudent to carry out densitometry even in healthy premenopausal women so that a diagnosis of osteopenia, if present, may be made. Admittedly, treatment may not be immediately indicated save for adjustment to exercise and dietary calcium, but the patient may be alerted to the need for future densitometric review at menopause when a critical decision on the use and duration of HRT may be made.

BONE PROTECTION AND OESTROGEN IN YOUNGER WOMEN

The general rules for the clinical use of oestrogen in the postmenopause apply with equal force to younger women. The practitioner should be satisfied that a valid indication exists and, usually, that circulating oestradiol is low (<150 pmol/l) in the presence of elevated levels of follicle stimulating hormone and luteinizing hormone (>25 IU/l). Pretreatment clinical checks must include breast and pelvic examinations and a measurement of blood pressure. The route of delivery is not critical for bone protection and may be oral, transdermal or subcutaneous. In general terms younger women need more daily oestrogen than do older women, and practitioners should not hesitate to use the higher dose regimens such as 1.25 mg of Premarin daily or the 100 μg patch. The patient should be carefully appraised of the early side-effects of oestrogen replacement, such as breast tenderness and appetite rise, and should be critically reviewed at 3 months. Thereafter a 6-monthly review is adequate with densitometry being repeated at 1 year to confirm that bone loss has been arrested. Management should exclude ascertainment that the patient is receiving at least 1000 mg calcium daily from her diet and that she has a reasonable exercise profile.

CONCLUSIONS

Osteoporosis is not exclusively a disease of the postmenopause. The disease has many antecedents and the mineral density of a bone, the main determinant of fracture risk, is a reflection of both hereditary and numerous environmental influences.

All women sustain a midlife menopause. They lose, due to oocyte exhaustion, the cyclic endogenous delivery of oestrogen, now known to be a central hormone in maintenance of bone density. Thus in younger women it is vital to identify, counsel and treat any who may be placed at a disadvantage in respect of bone strength – before the menopause approaches. The primary care team, the gynaecologist and the physician are best placed to supply access to the diagnostic techniques necessary to inform treatment. It is incumbent on all Health Authorities to make a densitometric service available at the general hospital level, so that patients at risk – or suspected to be at risk – may have their liability to fracture properly quantified and effectively managed.

REFERENCES

1. Consensus Development Conference (1991). Diagnosis, prophylaxis and treatment of osteoporosis. *Am. J. Med.,* **90**, 107–10
2. WHO Technical Report No 843 (1994). Assessment of fracture risk and its application to screening. (Geneva: World Health Organization)
3. Ott, S.M. (1990). Attainment of peak bone mass. *J. Clin. Endocrinol. Metab.,* **71**, 1082A–94A
4. Heaney, R.P. and Skillman, T.G. (1971). Calcium Metabolism in normal human pregnancy. *J. Clin. Endocrinol. Metab.,* **33**, 661–70
5. Tylavsky, F.A., Bortz, A.D., Hancock, R.L. and Anderson, J.J.B. (1989). Familial resemblance of radial bone mass between premenopausal mothers and their college-age daughters. *Calcif. Tissue Int.,* **45**, 265–72
6. Slemenda, C.W., Christian, J.C., Williams, C.J., Norton, J.A. and Johnston, C.C. (1991). Genetic determinants of bone mass in adult women: a re-evaluation of the twin model and the potential importance of gene interaction on heritability estimates. *J. Bone Miner. Res.,* **6**, 561–7
7. Johnston, C.C., Miller, J.Z., Slemenda, C.W., Reister, P.H.T.K., Siu Hui, M.S., Christian, J.C. and Peacock, M. (1992). Calcium supplementation and increases in bone mineral density in children. *N. Engl. J. Med.,* **327**, 82–7
8. Slemenda, C.W., Miller, J.Z., Hui, L.S., Reister, T.K. and Johnstone, C.C. (1991). Role of physical activity in development of skeletal mass in children. *J. Bone Miner. Res.,* **6**, 1227–33
9. Davies, M.C., Hall, M.L. and Jacobs, H.S. (1990). Bone mineral loss in young women with amenorrhoea. *Br. Med. J.,* **301**, 790–3
10. American Psychiatric Association (1993). Practice guidelines for eating disorders. *Am. J. Psychiatry,* **150**, 207–28
11. Kaplan, F.S., Pertschuk, M., Fallon, M. and Haddad, J. (1985). Osteoporosis and hip fracture in a young woman with anorexia nervosa. *Clin. Orthop. Rel. Res.,* **212**, 250–54
12. Klibanski, A., Biller, B.M.K., Schoenfeld, D.A., Herzog, D.B. and Saxe, V.C. (1995). The effects of estrogen administration on trabecular bone loss in young women with anorexia nervosa. *J. Clin. Endocrinol. Metab.,* **80**, 898–904.
13. Koppelman, M.C.S., Kurtz, D.W. and Morrish, K.A. (1984). Vertebral body bone mineral content in hyperprolactinemic women. *J. Clin. Endocrinol. Metab.,* **59**, 1050–3
14. Schlechte, J., Walkner, L. and Kathol, M. (1992). A longitudinal analysis of premenopausal bone loss in healthy women and women with hyperprolactinaemia. *J. Clin. Endocrinol. Metab.,* **75**, 698–703

15. Klibanski, A., Biller, B.M.K., Rosenthal, D.I., Schoenfeld, D.A. and Saxe, V. (1988). Effects of prolactin and estrogen deficiency in amenorrheic bone loss. *J. Clin. Endocrinol. Metab.*, **67**, 124–30
16. Biller, B.M.K., Baum, H.B.A., Rosenthal, D.I., Saxe, V.C., Charpie, P.M. and Klibanski, A. (1992). Progressive trabecular osteopenia in women with hyperprolactinemic amenorrhea. *J. Clin. Endocrinol. Metab.*, **75**, 692–7
17. Marcus, R., Cann, C. and Madvig, P. (1985). Menstrual function and bone in women distance runners, endocrine and metabolic features. *Ann. Intern. Med.*, **102**, 158–63
18. Lloyd, T., Myers, C., Buchanan, J.R. and Demers, L.M. (1988). Collegiate women athletes with irregular menses during adolescence have decreased bone density. *Obstet. Gynecol.*, **72**, 639–42
19. Wolman, R.L., Faulmann, L. and Clark, P. (1991). Different training patterns and bone mineral density in elite female athletes. *Ann. Rheum. Diseases*, **50**, 487–9
20. Myburgh, K.H., Hutchins, J., Fataar, A.B., Hough, S.F. and Noakes, T.D. (1990). Low bone density is an etiologic factor for stress fractures in athletes. *Ann. Intern. Med.*, **113**, 754–9
21. Matta, W.H., Shaw, R.W., Hesp, R. and Evans, R. (1988). Reversible trabecular bone density loss following induced hypo-estrogenism with the GnRH analogue buserelin in premenopausal women. *Clin. Endocrinol. (Oxf.)*, **29**, 45–51
22. Shaw, R.W. (1994). A risk benefit assessment of drugs used in the treatment of endometriosis. *Drug Safety*, **11**, 104–13
23. Purdie, D.W., Aaron, J.E. and Selby, P.L. (1988). Bone histology and mineral homeostasis in human pregnancy. *Br. J. Obstet. Gynaecol.*, **95**, 849–54
24. Sowers, M., Cortan, G. and Shapiro, B. (1993). Changes in bone density with lactation. *J. Am. Med. Assoc.*, **269**, 3130–5
25. Cummings, S.R., Black, D.M. and Nevitt, M.C. (1993). Bone density at various sites for prediction of hip fractures. *Lancet*, **341**, 72–5
26. Felson, D.T., Zhang, Y., Hannan, M.T., Kiel, D.P., Wilson, W.F. and Anderson, J.J. (1993). The effect of postmenopausal estrogen therapy on bone density in elderly women. *N. Engl. J. Med.*, **329**, 1141–6
27. Anwerx, J. and Bouillon, R. (1986). Mineral and bone metabolism in thyroid disease: a review. *Q. J. Med.*, New Series, **60**, 737–52
28. McDermott, M.T., Kidd, G.S., Blue, P., Ghaed, V. and Hofeldt, F.D. (1983). Reduced bone mineral content in totally thyroidectomized patients. Possible effect of calcitonin deficiency. *J. Clin. Endocrinol. Metab.*, **56**, 936–9

29. Heath, H., Melton., L.J. and Chu, C.P. (1980). Diabetes mellitus and risk of skeletal fracture. *N. Engl. J. Med.*, **303**, 567–70

30. Raskin, P., Stevenson, M.R.M., Barilla, D.E. and Pak, C.Y.C. (1978). The hypercalciuria of diabetes mellitus; its amelioration with insulin. *Clin. Endocrinol.*, **9**, 329–35

31. Johnston, C.C., Hui, S.L. and Longcope, C. (1985). Bone mass and sex steroid concentrations in postmenopausal Caucasian diabetics. *Metabolism*, **34**, 544–50

32. Deutsch, S. and Benjamin, F. (1978). Effect of diabetic status on fractionated estrogen levels in postmenopausal women. *J. Am. Obstet. Gynecol.*, **130**, 105–6

33. Duncan, H. (1972). Osteoporosis in rheumatoid arthritis and corticosteroid induced osteoporosis. Symposium on metabolic bone disease. *Orthop. Clin. North Am.*, **3**, 571–83

34. Scame, J.L., Sebert, J.L. and Delcambre, B. (1979). L'ostéoporose cortisonique. *Nouv. Presse Med.*, **8**, 1675–80

35. Seeman, E., Melton, L.J. III, O'Fallon, W.M. and Riggs, B.L. (1983). Risk factors for spinal osteoporosis in men. *Am. J. Med.*, **75**, 977–83

36. Cann, C.E., Martin, M.C., Genant, H.K. and Jaffe, R.B. (1984) Decreased spinal mineral content in amenorrheic women. *J. Am. Med. Assoc.*, **251**, 626–9

37. Watson, N.R., Studd, J.W.W., Garnet, T., Savvas, M. and Milligan, P. (1995). Bone loss after hysterectomy with ovarian conservation. *Obstet. Gynecol.*, **86**, 72–7

38. Kahn, S.A., Pace, J.E., Cox, M.L., Cox, S.A.L. and Hodkinson, H.M. (1994) Osteoporosis and genetic influence: a three-generation study. *Postgrad. Med. J.*, **70**, 798–800

8

What's new in hormone replacement therapy?

D.H. Barlow

INTRODUCTION

This symposium has been concerned with many of the adverse consequences of hypo-oestrogenic states and their management. Oestrogen replacement is well known to counter many of the problems and has been available to women for decades. Despite this the issues surrounding the use of hormone replacement therapy (HRT) are much more complex than any simplistic assumption that those affected by the effects of hypo-oestrogenism will necessarily wish to use HRT, or that the forms of HRT available are all that could be wished.

There is considerable survey evidence which demonstrates that the uptake of HRT by women in the perimenopause and post-menopause is generally below 20% in the UK and there is some evidence that the use of HRT has been of relatively limited duration when used in non-hysterectomized women[1]. The basis for this pattern of use is complex. The influences on decision-making in relation to starting HRT are demonstrated in two studies which employed a similar methodology. These assessed the attitudes of women in Iowa, USA[2] and in Aberdeen[3] which examined the influences on a woman deciding to start HRT. The findings of both studies were similar. Important positive influences were the good experience of a friend or the recommendation of a doctor. Negative influences were the bad experience of a friend and concern about cancer. Another strongly negative factor was the expectation of withdrawal bleeding.

In another study, by Wren and Brown[4], dissatisfaction with menstruation was a prominent factor. The problem of achieving good compliance with HRT regimens is currently of great interest in the light of reports that many women fail to initiate prescribed therapy or soon discontinue it[5] even where there has been a recommendation that reduced bone density justifies HRT use[6,7]. The potential importance of achieving good rates of continuation of HRT is reinforced by evidence that both skeletal and cardiovascular benefit may be significantly eroded once the HRT is discontinued. There is evidence to suggest that by the time women who used HRT after the menopause have lost most of the skeletal advantage gained are approaching 80 years, the age range at which hip fracture is most likely to occur[8] they have lost most of the skeletal advantage gained. Similarly, some of the non-lipid mechanisms which may be responsible for the beneficial effect of HRT on cardiovascular disease[9,10] are likely to have their action mainly during the use of HRT. These data emphasize the importance of developing forms of HRT which may be acceptable for long-term use by women from the time of menopause or by more elderly women when they have reached the age when fractures and heart disease are more likely to occur.

THE IMPORTANCE OF SAFETY

In the development of HRT regimens the guiding principles must be to maximize safety whilst maintaining efficacy. The focus of safety has to be wide because of the diverse range of potential problems which have to be considered. Some of these are a direct, but inappropriate, extrapolation from the evidence concerning oral contraception. Since the majority of regimens available have been oestrogen only or opposed formulations involving cyclical progestogen the safety data has largely related to these. Hypertension does not appear to be an issue with HRT[11,12], nor is there good evidence for a significant increase in the risk of venous thrombosis in HRT users[13]. With cyclical opposed HRT the risk of endometrial cancer is

118

not significantly higher than in untreated women[14] whereas the risk of endometrial cancer is elevated and remains so for years after cessation of unopposed oestrogen treatment[15]. The risk of breast cancer is the most controversial issue and although the literature is generally reassuring there is some degree of disagreement in the meta-analyses which have been reported. Steinberg and co-workers[16] have indicated no increase in risk until after at least 5 years use and with a 30% increase in risk after 15 years use. In contrast Dupont and Page[17] did not find a duration of use effect and similarly Colditz and colleagues[18] found no duration of use effect but an increase in risk with current use. Decisions about whether to use HRT and for how long, particularly in more 'at risk' subgroups, must be weighed by the individual woman in consultation with her professional advisors.

EFFICACY

Efficacy is difficult to define since the HRT can address several end points of benefit to the woman. It is likely that the various potential oestrogen preparations achieve similar levels of efficacy when equivalent doses are delivered. Indeed it is more likely that individual variations will be a more important factor influencing the efficacy than the preparation chosen. Where the end point of interest is symptom relief the efficacy of a preparation can be directly studied in prospective randomized therapeutic trials. However, with oestrogen there are other efficacy end points which cannot realistically be tested in prospective studies and depend on epidemiological evidence. The most prominent of these are the effect of HRT on the prevention of osteoporotic fracture and the prevention of coronary heart disease. With the bone effect there is the surrogate measure of bone density which correlates with fracture risk but it is not an ideal measure, particularly if the studies are of relatively short duration. In such studies of just 1 or 2 years the short-term effects on bone turnover are associated with such reactionary changes in the balance of bone formation and resorption that it is difficult to predict the effect of the chronic use of the preparation over several years, the duration of therapy intended for worthwhile alleviation of osteoporotic fracture risk. With coronary heart disease the lipid-related surrogate end points are less closely linked to the risk of myocardial infarction so that it is even more difficult to test the efficacy of a specific oestrogen than with bone.

NEW DEVELOPMENTS IN OESTROGEN PREPARATIONS

Although the large amount of literature on efficacy and safety is based largely on the study of conjugated oestrogens in American women and Swedish data on oestradiol valerate, one theme in recent work has been the continuing expansion of alternatives to oral oestrogen.

Alcohol-based patches have been available for many years but now we are seeing a worthwhile expansion of the availability of matrix patches beyond the single 50 µg dose 'Evorel' patch which has been available for the past couple of years. British doctors can now choose from a range of Evorel doses (25 µg to 100 µg) and the 'Fematrix' 80 µg matrix patch. The competing patches have similar duration of action and monthly cost but claim different rates of skin reaction and adhesiveness so that women who wish to use oestrogen patches have a range of options. The percutaneous oestradiol gel, 'Estrogel', has now been added to this range of transdermal oestrogen skin patches.

'Estrogel' is a water-soluble gel containing oestradiol in alcohol. The gel is applied to the skin once daily over an area of at least 700 cm^2 to deliver 750 µg oestradiol in 1.25 g of gel. The recommended dose is between 1.5 and 3.0 mg daily. The gel has been available in France for more than a decade and in France it is a leading oestrogen preparation where it is provided as a simple tube from which the gel is squeezed, the amount being measured against a plastic spatula ruler which is provided. The British presentation is in a metered dose dispenser. Two measures from the metered dose dispenser are equivalent to one length measured against the French plastic spatula (2.5 g gel or 1.5 mg oestradiol). The oestradiol is delivered to the skin for a period of approximately 3 min but further delivery ceases when the ethanol carrier has evaporated. The skin is then dry and non-greasy. Immediate washing may remove some of the dose but after 30 min to 1 h the delivered dose cannot be removed.

Oestradiol patches and gel are alternatives to oral oestrogen for systemic therapy but, in addition, there have been developments in the local delivery of oestrogen where the intention is to avoid systemic therapy. This approach is aimed at the treatment and prevention of urogenital atrophy (UGA) which may be associated with both symptoms of vaginal atrophy, irritation and dyspareunia[19] and urinary symptoms such as frequency of micturition and some cases of urinary incontinence[20,21]. The atrophic genital symptoms often improve in response to local oestrogen, however, the response of urinary incontinence, which is often subjectively improved, is less predictable in terms of objective measures and the literature is inconsistent[22]. Local vaginal therapy has been developed beyond the use of creams, which have the disadvantage of being messy, through waxy pessaries to a long-acting vaginal tablet 'Vagifem' introduced a couple of years ago[23] and an oestradiol-releasing vaginal ring recently introduced known as 'Estring'. The 'Vagifem' vaginal tablet provides 25 µg oestradiol and is inserted vaginally twice weekly. In a prospective randomized placebo-controlled study the percentage of women experiencing moderate or severe vaginal atrophy symptoms was reduced from 78.8% to 10.7%, over 12 weeks, whereas in the placebo treated group the equivalent percentages were 81.9% and 29.9%, respectively[23]. The more recently introduced option is the oestradiol-releasing ring 'Estring' which is a soft ring with a diameter of 55 mm. The ring releases 5–10 µg oestradiol daily and remains in the vagina for 3 months when it is then replaced. This implies an annual oestradiol dose of only 3.5 mg. As with the vaginal tablet the systemic effect is negligible and there is no detectable endometrial proliferation[24]. The ring was reported to induce a significant improvement in vaginal indices and in the clinical assessment of the vaginal mucosa. There was also a significant improvement in symptoms of urogenital atrophy with cure or improvement reported by more than 90% of women[24].

OESTROGEN AND PROGESTOGEN COMBINED REGIMENS

Monthly cyclical regimens

The role of progestogens in HRT developed as a direct result of the adverse data on endometrial-cancer risk published in the mid-1970s[25,26]. The formulation regimens which resulted employed 7 days then 10 or 12 days progestogen administered cyclically per month. These regimens appear to have provided the long-term safety which was hoped for in the prevention of endometrial hyperplasia and cancer[14]. The range of progestogens employed was for many years limited to the two 19-nortestosterone derivatives, norethisterone and norgestrel/levonorgestrel, but less androgenic progestogens have become available for use in HRT more recently so that clinicians can offer women cyclical regimens involving dydrogesterone or medroxyprogesterone acetate, however, combined cyclical preparations are not yet available but should soon further extend the range of options as combined oestrogen and progestogen packs. The low doses at which progestogens are used in HRT regimens mean that for many women the fact that the progestogens most commonly prescribed are androgenic is not a significant issue, however, for a minority the androgenic progestogens do induce premenstrual syndrome-like side-effects. In addition, it has been a concern that the lipid effects of the androgenic progestogens might be negating a significant proportion of the lipid benefit induced by the oestrogen[27]. Despite this concern there is biochemical evidence that androgenic progestogens need not have an adverse lipid effect[28] and there is growing evidence that the lipid effects of HRT are only one of several beneficial effects mediated by oestrogen[29] and epidemiological evidence also supports the overall effect of androgenic progestogens in HRT to be beneficial[30]. Whatever the overall contribution of the lipid effect of HRT we do have evidence that the non-androgenic progestogens optimize the impact on high-density lipoprotein (HDL) cholesterol[31-33].

Recent data concerning the clinical management of cyclical regimens include evidence that the timing of the regular withdrawal bleed is not a guide to the risk of endometrial hyperplasia. There was evidence that an early onset of the withdrawal bleed during the progestogen phase of the HRT indicated a risk of incomplete secretory transformation and, by implication, an increased risk of developing hyperplasia[34]. Recent data, from a much larger study, have shown that modern cyclical regimens are associated with a hyperplasia rate of 2–3% and that the pattern of onset of bleeding does not predict the cases with hyperplasia[35].

In considering recent developments in HRT there are a number of themes to consider of which the most important is likely to be the newer regimens which aim to minimize the experience of vaginal bleeding. These approaches can be divided into those (1) which aim to provide endometrial safety but without using progestogens every month and those (2) which provide frequent or continuous progestogen with the aim of inducing a bleed free state.

Long-cycle regimens

Infrequent exposure to progestogen during continuing exposure to oestrogen has attracted interest with 3-, 4- and 6-monthly exposure patterns having been explored. The longest interval between progestogen courses, at 6 months, has been reported by Kemp and colleagues[36] who demonstrated that good compliance could be achieved with a continuation rate above 90%. Over 4 years there were no endometrial malignancies but two cases of atypical hyperplasia developed in a study of 85 women. In a study of 4-monthly progestogen administration, again good control of bleeding was achieved in the 3 months in which the oestrogen (oestradiol 2 mg) was administered continuously without progestogen[37]. In the fourth cycle norethisterone 1 mg was given for 10 days. This study involved more than 1000 women of whom 528 agreed to 6-monthly hysteroscopy and biopsy and 50 women in a pilot group agreed to monthly hysteroscopy and biopsy over 16 months. This intensive investigation demonstrated that after 3 months of continuous oestrogen there is a 13 to 17% rate of hyperplasia, but that after the progestogen course in the fourth cycles (cycles 4, 8, 12 and 16) hyperplasia is not detected.

The infrequent progestogen regimen which has reached licensing for use in the UK has the name 'Tridestra' and is oestradiol valerate

(2 mg) for 84 days in 3 months with medroxyprogesterone acetate (20 mg) for the last 14 days of oestrogen. Studies of this regimen indicate that the risk of endometrial hyperplasia is low. Hirvonen and co-workers[38] reported one case of adenomatous hyperplasia in a series of 227 women completing 1 year of therapy in a study with a high 1-year continuation rate of 86%. In another study Koskela and colleagues[39] reported no hyperplasia cases in a series of 30 women. Since the regimen is oestrogen alone for most of the time good efficacy in terms of symptoms and systemic effects on bone and the cardiovascular system are to be expected; whereas the more uncertain question relates to the control of the endometrial bleeding pattern. Crona and co-workers[40] have reported that this regimen gives a similar rate of unscheduled bleeding to a continuous combined HRT regimen, with 54% and 57%, respectively, reporting unscheduled bleeding during the 1st year of treatment. Hirvonen and colleagues[38] have reported that the unscheduled bleeding decreases with time, with most women settling to an expected 3-monthly bleed. The average day of onset of the bleed has been shown to be day 86[39].

Bleed-free regimens

The cyclophasic approach

There are two approaches to bleed-free regimens. Easily the most widely used is the continuous use of oestrogen and progestogen together as a 'continuous combined' regimen. The other approach is less well established and involves the continuous administration of oestrogen and the use of progestogen for 3 days out of every 6. This latter approach has been named 'cyclophasic' HRT.

Cyclophasic HRT has been reported to provide amenorrhoea after initial phase in which vaginal bleeding or spotting can occur. In the published study the progestogen was 0.35 mg norethisterone given for 3 out of every 6 days whilst piperazine oestrone sulphate (0.75 mg) was given continuously[41]. Forty women were studied of whom 80% had no bleeding by 6 months. There was good compliance with 83% completing 24 months. The regimen effectively prevented endometrial hyperplasia and good symptom control was achieved. The only lipid effects were small rises in high-density lipoprotein cholesterol and triglycerides at 24 months[41]. During the first few months on this regimen, bleeding is not predictable, although generally not excessive. Further studies are required before the validity of this approach will be clear.

The continuous combined approach

The use of regimens offering bleed-free therapy is not entirely new to the UK since tibolone has been available for several years and offers a single molecule with oestrogenic and progestogenic properties so that a continuous oestrogen and progestogen effect is achieved with amenorrhoea as the aim. Although continuous combined HRT can be considered to aim at the same end point by the similar means of providing continuous oestrogenic and progestogenic stimulation, it might be considered to carry the advantage that the components involved are more well-defined hormonal entities than tibolone. Continuous combined HRT has been available, licensed in some European countries, for several years but the first licensed preparation became available in the UK only in 1995. This was 'Kliofem' which combines continuous oestradiol valerate (2 mg) and norethisterone (1 mg). There is now a considerable experience of this preparation with long-term data available on its metabolic effects and bleeding patterns and efficacy suggesting a performance comparable with cyclical HRT except for the likelihood that amenorrhoea will result[42–44]. Other continuous combined HRT regimens have now been explored, including the use of desogestrel[45,46], dydrogesterone[47] and medroxyprogesterone acetate[48–50]. It is likely that there will be a range of different continuous combined HRT regimens available in the future. There is a widespread perception that this style of regimen will become the standard for women who are already menopausal and who wish to continue with HRT for a reasonable time. The use of these regimens in women who are still perimenopausal is associated with an unacceptably high risk of unpredictable bleeding.

INTRAUTERINE PROGESTOGEN DELIVERY

An alternative approach to bleed-free HRT regimens is to provide a continuous combined regimen by delivering the progestogen directly to the uterine cavity by means of a progestogen-releasing intrauterine contraceptive device. The device, which has been developed in Scandinavia, is now available in the UK for use in contraception and releases levonorgestrel into the uterine cavity over 3 to 5 years with minimal systemic effect. Nilsson and colleagues[51] have demonstrated that the endometrial concentration of levonorgestrel is much higher with this device (468–1568 ng/g wet-weight tissue) than with oral levonorgestrel (2.8–4.2 ng/g wet-weight tissue). The endometrial effect has been shown to be that of inducing epithelial gland atrophy and a decidualized stroma. Potential uses for this device, not yet licensed in the UK, are in the management of menorrhagia where dramatic reductions in blood losses are reported[52,53], endometrial hyperplasia where it provides a potent stimulus to reverse hyperplasia[54] and as a progestogen in HRT where the woman achieves a likelihood of amenorrhoea and contraception but a low risk of systemic progestogenic symptom or metabolic effects[55,56]. This method of progestogen delivery has been shown to provide better endometrial control than long-acting progestogen implants[57].

CONCLUSION

As stated at the beginning of this presentation, 1995 has seen a significant expansion of the range of licensed HRT options available. These have included several new preparations which offer something significantly different from what was previously available. In the past it has been possible for a doctor to be familiar with possibly one oral cyclical regimen and a patch regimen and feel that alternative preparations were not substantially different. The option developments described in this presentation include a number of regimens which offer significantly different choices to women. It may take doctors, not familiar with these developments, a little time to assimilate them but it is clear that the field of HRT is now more diverse that ever before and therefore it is much more likely that a woman who wants to use HRT may find a regimen which suits her for her stage of life.

REFERENCES

1. Barlow, D.H., Grosset, K.A., Hart, H. and Hart, D.M. (1989). A study of the experience of Glasgow women in the climacteric years. *Br. J. Obstet. Gynaecol.*, **96**, 1192–7

2. Ferguson, K.J., Hoegh, C. and Johnson, S. (1989) Estrogen replacement therapy. A survey of women's knowledge and attitudes. *Arch. Intern. Med.*, **149**, 133–6

3. Sinclair, H.K., Bond, C.M. and Taylor, R.J. (1993). Hormone replacement therapy: a study of women's knowledge and attitudes. *Br. J. Gen. Pract.*, **43**, 365–70

4. Wren, B.G. and Brown, L. (1990). Compliance with hormonal replacement therapy. *Maturitas*, **13**, 17–21

5. Ravnikar, V.A. (1987). Compliance with hormone therapy. *Am. J. Obstet. Gynecol.*, **156**, 1332–4

6. Marsh, M.S., Stevenson, J.C. and Whitehead, M.I. (1993). Compliance with hormone replacement therapy (HRT) after screening for post menopausal osteoporosis. *Br. J. Obstet. Gynaecol.*, **100**, 399–400

7. Ryan, P.J., Harrison, R., Blake, G.M. and Fogelman, I. (1992). Compliance with hormone replacement therapy (HRT) after screening for post menopausal osteoporosis. *Br. J. Obstet. Gynaecol.*, **99**, 325–8

8. Felson, D.T., Zhang, Y., Hannan, M.T. and Anderson, J.J. (1993). Effects of weight and body mass index on bone mineral density in men and women: the Framingham study. *J. Bone Miner. Res.*, **8**, 567–73

9. Collins, P., Rosano, G.M., Jiang, C., Lindsay, D., Sarrel, P.M. and Poole Wilson, P.A. (1993). Cardiovascular protection by oestrogen–a calcium antagonist effect? *Lancet*, **341**, 1264–5

10. Hillard, T.C., Bourne, T.H., Whitehead, M.I., Crayford, T.B., Collins, W.P. and Campbell, S. (1992). Differential effects of transdermal estradiol and sequential progestogens on impedance to flow within the uterine arteries of postmenopausal women. *Fertil. Steril.*, **58**, 959–63

11. Hassager, C., Riis, B.J., Strom, V., Guyene, T.T. and Christiansen, C. (1987). The long-term effect of oral and percutaneous estradiol on plasma renin substrate and blood pressure. *Circulation*, **76,** 753–8

12. Lip, G.Y., Beevers, M., Churchill, D., and Beevers, D.G. (1994). Hormone replacement therapy and blood pressure in hypertensive women. *J. Hum. Hypertens.*, **8**, 491–4

13. Young, R.L., Goepfert, A.R. and Goldzieher, H.W. (1991). Estrogen replacement therapy is not conducive of venous thromboembolism. *Maturitas*, **13**, 189–92

14. Persson, I., Adami, H.O., Bergkvist, L., Lindgren, A., Pettersson, B., Hoover, R. and Schairer, C. (1989). Risk of endometrial cancer after treatment with oestrogens alone or in conjunction with progestogens: results of a prospective study. *Br. Med. J.*, **298**, 147–51

15. Paganini-Hill, A., Ross, R.K. and Henderson, B.E. (1989). Endometrial cancer and patterns of use of oestrogen replacement therapy: a cohort study. *Br. J. Cancer*, **59**, 445–7

16. Steinberg, K.K., Thacker, S.B., Smith, S.J., Stroup, D.F., Zack, M.M., Flanders, W.D. and Berkelman, R.L. (1991). A meta-analysis of the effect of estrogen replacement therapy on the risk of breast cancer. *J. Am. Med. Assoc.*, **265**, 1985–90

17. Dupont, W.D. and Page, D.L. (1991). Menopausal estrogen replacement therapy and breast cancer. *Arch. Intern. Med.*, **151**, 67–72

18. Colditz, G.A., Egan, K.M. and Stampfer, M.J. (1993). Hormone replacement therapy and risk of breast cancer: results from epidemiologic studies. *Am. J. Obstet. Gynecol.*, **168**, 1473–80

19. Semmens, J.P. and Wagner, G. (1982). Estrogen deprivation and vaginal function in postmenopausal women. *J. Am. Med. Assoc.*, **248**, 445–8

20. Molander, U. (1993). Urinary incontinence and related urogenital symptoms in elderly women. *Acta Obstet. Gynecol. Scand.*, **158** (Suppl.), 1–22

21. Rekers, H., Drogendijk, A.C., Valkenburg, H.A. and Riphagen, F. (1992). The menopause, urinary incontinence and other symptoms of the genito-urinary tract. *Maturitas*, **15**, 101–11

22. Fantl, J.A., Wyman, J.F., Anderson, R.L., Matt, D.W. and Bump, R.C. (1988). Postmenopausal urinary incontinence: comparison between non-estrogen-supplemented and estrogen-supplemented women. *Obstet. Gynecol.*, **71**, 823–8

23. Eriksen, P.S. and Rasmussen, H. (1992). Low-dose 17 beta-estradiol vaginal tablets in the treatment of atrophic vaginitis: a double-blind placebo controlled study. *Eur. J. Obstet. Gynecol. Reprod. Biol.*, **44**, 137–44

24. Smith, P., Heimer, G., Lindskog, M. and Ulmsten, U. (1993). Oestradiol-releasing vaginal ring for treatment of postmenopausal urogenital atrophy. *Maturitas*, **16**, 145–54

25. Ziel, H.K. and Finkle, W.D. (1975). Increased risk of endometrial carcinoma among users of conjugated estrogens. *N. Engl. J. Med.*, **293**, 1167–70

26. Smith, D.C., Prentice, R., Thompson, D.J. and Herrmann, W.L. (1975). Association of exogenous estrogen and endometrial carcinoma. *N. Engl. J. Med.*, **293**, 1164–7

27. Barrett Connor, E. (1993). Estrogen and estrogen-progestogen replacement: therapy and cardiovascular diseases. *Am. J. Med.*, **95**, 40S–3S

28. Farish E., Fletcher, C.D., Hart, D.M., Teo, H.T., Alazzawi, F. and Howie, C. (1986). The effects of conjugated equine oestrogens with and without a cyclical progestogen on lipoproteins, and HDL subfractions in postmenopausal women. *Acta Endocrinol. Copenh.*, **113**, 123–7

29. Gangar, K.F., Reid, B.A., Crook, D., Hillard, T.C. and Whitehead, M.I. (1993). Oestrogens and atherosclerotic vascular disease – local vascular factors. *Baillieres Clin. Endocrinol. Metab.*, **7**, 47–59

30. Falkeborn, M., Persson, I., Adami, H.O., Bergstrom, R., Eaker, E., Lithell, H., Mohsen, R. and Naessen, T. (1992). The risk of acute myocardial infarction after oestrogen and oestrogen-progestogen replacement. *Br. J. Obstet. Gynaecol.*, **99**, 821–8

31. van der Mooren, M.J., Demacker, P.N., Thomas, C.M., Borm, G.F. and Rolland, R. (1993). A 2-year study on the beneficial effects of 17 beta-oestradiol-dydrogesterone therapy on serum lipoproteins and Lp(a) in postmenopausal women: no additional unfavourable effects of dydrogesterone. *Eur. J. Obstet. Gynecol. Reprod. Biol.*, **52**, 117–23

32. Fletcher, C.D., Farish, E., Dagen, M.M., Alazzawi, F., McQueen, D. and Hart, D.M. (1988). The effects of conjugated equine estrogens plus cyclical dydrogesterone on serum lipoproteins and apoproteins in postmenopausal women. *Acta Endocrinol. Copenh.*, **117**, 339–42

33. The Writing Group for the PEPI Trial (1995). Effects of estrogen or estrogen/progestin regimens on heart disease risk factors in postmenopausal women. The Postmenopausal Estrogen/Progestin Interventions (PEPI) Trial. *J. Am. Med. Assoc.*, **273**, 199–208

34. Padwick, M., Pryse-Davies, J. and Whitehead, M.I. (1986). A simple method for determining the optimal dosage of progestin in postmenopausal women receiving estrogens. *N. Engl. J. Med.*, **315**, 930–4

35. Sturdee, D.W., Barlow, D.H., Ulrich, L.G., Wells, M., Gydesen, H., Campbell, M., O'Brien, K. and Vessey, M. (1994). Is the timing of withdrawal bleeding a guide to endometrial safety during sequential oestrogen-progestagen replacement therapy? UK Continuous Combined HRT Study Investigators. *Lancet*, **344**, 979–82

36. Kemp, J.F., Fryer, J.A. and Baber, R.J. (1989) An alternative regimen of hormone replacement therapy to improve patient compliance. *Aust. NZ J. Obstet. Gynaecol.*, **29**, 66–9

37. David, A., Czernobilsky, B. and Weisglass, L. (1994). Long-cyclic hormonal cycle therapy in postmenopausal women. In Berg, G. and Hammer, M. (eds.) *The Modern Management of the Menopause Proceedings of the Seventh International Congress on the Menopause*, pp.463–70. (London: Parthenon Publishing)

38. Hirvonen, E., Salmi, T. and Puojakka, J. (1992). Three-months estrogen/progestogen treatment regimen in postmenopausal hormone replacement. *Proceedings of the Congress of European Association of Gynaecologists and Obstetricians*, Helsinki, Finland, abstr.

39. Koskela, J., Wilen-Rosenqvist, C., Vartiainen, E. and Hirvonen, E. (1990). Three-monthly sequential oestradiol/medroxyprogesterone acetate (MPA) treatment regimen in postmenopausal women. *Proceedings of the Sixth International Congress on the Menopause*, October 1990, Bangkok, Thailand, abstr. 84

40. Crona, N., Lindhe, B., Cavalli-Bjorkman, B., Einerth, Y., Jorgensen, O.H., Nordenstrom, S., Sandstedt, B., Velinder-Klacker, G.M. and Astrom, G. (1990). Effects of two oestrogen and progestogen combinations on climacteric symptoms, bleeding patterns and the endometrium. *Proceedings of the Sixth International Congress on the Menopause*, October 1990, Bangkok, Thailand, abstr. 193

41. Casper, R.F. and Chapdelaine, A. (1993). Estrogen and interrupted progestin: a new concept for menopausal hormone replacement therapy. *Am. J. Obstet. Gynecol.*, **168**, 1188–94

42. Staland, B. (1981). Continuous treatment with natural oestrogens and progestogens. A method to avoid endometrial stimulation. *Maturitas*, **3**, 145–56

43. Christiansen, C. and Riis, B.J. (1990). Five years with continuous combined oestrogen/progestogen therapy. Effects on calcium metabolism, lipoproteins, and bleeding pattern. *Br. J. Obstet. Gynaecol.*, **97**, 1087–92

44. Munk Jensen, N., Ulrich, L.G., Obel, E.B., Nielsen, S.P., Edwards. D. and Meinertz, H. (1994). Continuous combined and sequential estradiol and norethindrone acetate treatment of postmenopausal women: effect of plasma lipoproteins in a two-year placebo-controlled trial. *Am. J. Obstet. Gynecol.*, **171**, 132–8

45. Marsh, M.S., Crook, D., Lees, B., Worthington, M., Ellerington, M., Whitcroft, S., Whitehead, M.I. and Stevenson, J.C. (1993). The effects of oral desogestrel and estradiol continuous combined hormone

replacement therapy on serum lipids and body composition in post-menopausal women. *Basic Life Sci.*, **60**, 219–20

46. Marsh, M.S., Crook. D., Whitcroft, S.I., Worthington, M., Whitehead, M.I. and Stevenson, J.C. (1994). Effect of continuous combined estrogen and desogestrel hormone replacement therapy on serum lipids and lipoproteins. *Obstet. Gynecol.*, **83**, 19–23

47. Voetberg, G.A., Netelenbos, J.C., Kenemans, P., Peters Muller, E.R. and van de Weijer, P.H. (1994). Estrogen replacement therapy continuously combined with four different dosages of dydrogesterone: effect on calcium and lipid metabolism. *J. Clin. Endocrinol. Metab.*, **79**, 1465–9

48. Archer, D.F., Pickar, J.H. and Bottiglioni, F. (1994). Bleeding patterns in postmenopausal women taking continuous combined or sequential regimens of conjugated estrogens with medroxyprogesterone acetate. Menopause Study Group. *Obstet. Gynecol.*, **83**, 686–92

49. Grey, A.B., Cundy, T.F. and Reid, I.R. (1994). Continuous combined oestrogen/progestin therapy is well tolerated and increases bone density at the hip and spine in post-menopausal osteoporosis. *Clin. Endocrinol. Oxf.*, **40**, 671–7

50. Mattsson, L.A., Samsioe, G., von Schoultz, B., Uvebrant, M. and Wiklund, I. (1993). Transdermally administered oestradiol combined with oral medroxyprogesterone acetate: the effects on lipoprotein metabolism in postmenopausal women. *Br. J. Obstet. Gynaecol.*, **100,** 450–3

51. Nilsson, B., Sodergard, R., Damber, M.G. and von-Schoultz, B. (1982). Danazol and gestagen displacement of testosterone and influence on sex-hormone-binding globulin capacity. *Fertil. Steril.*, **38**, 48–53

52. Andersson, K. and Rybo, G. (1990). Levonorgestrel-releasing intrauterine device in the treatment of menorrhagia. *Br. J. Obstet. Gynaecol.*, **97**, 690–4

53. Milsom, I., Andersson, K., Andersch, B. and Rybo, G. (1991). A comparison of flurbiprofen, tranexamic acid, and a levonorgestrel-releasing intrauterine contraceptive device in the treatment of idiopathic menorrhagia. *Am. J. Obstet. Gynecol.*, **164**, 879–83

54. Scarselli, G., Tantini, C., Colafranceschi, M., Taddei, G.L., Bargelli, G., Venturini, N. and Branconi, F. (1988). Levo-norgestrel-nova-T and precancerous lesions of the endometrium. *Eur. J. Gynaecol. Oncol.*, **9**, 284–6

55. Andersson, K., Mattsson, L.A., Rybo, G. and Stadberg, E. (1992). Intrauterine release of levonorgestrel – a new way of adding progestogen in hormone replacement therapy. *Obstet. Gynecol.*, **79**, 963–7

56. Raudaskoski, T.H., Lahti, E.I., Kauppila, A.J., Apaja Sarkkinen, M.A. and Laatikainen, T.J. (1995). Transdermal estrogen with a levonorgestrel-

releasing intrauterine device for climacteric complaints: clinical and endometrial responses. *Am. J. Obstet. Gynecol.*, **172**, 114–19

57. Suhonen, S.P., Allonen, H.O. and Lahteenmaki, P. (1995). Sustained-release estradiol implants and a levonorgestrel-releasing intrauterine device in hormone replacement therapy. *Am. J. Obstet. Gynecol.*, **172**, 562–7

9

Risks of hormone replacement therapy

D. Ross

INTRODUCTION

Many of the commonly perceived risks of postmenopausal hormone replacement therapy (HRT), such as weight gain, hypertension and venous thromboembolism, are inappropriately extrapolated from data on combined oral contraceptives. There is a complete lack of epidemiological evidence associating these risks with HRT use, without doubt, due to the fact that the oestrogens used in HRT are of much lower potency than those (predominantly ethinyl oestradiol) found in combined oral contraceptives. Appreciation of the differences between these groups of hormonal preparations should enable most doctors to arrive at a practical approach to prescribing HRT for women who might previously have been denied it.

Of far more concern to the majority of women is the possibility of an increased risk of cancer, particularly breast cancer, with long-term use of HRT. The degree to which this concern influences women in their decisions about HRT is probably out of proportion to the numerical magnitude of any true effect, reflecting both the emotive nature of any discussion of cancer and the amount of media attention devoted to it. Counselling women about the possible long-term risks of HRT use is a difficult process, one which is not aided by the mass of apparently conflicting evidence and opinion that abounds.

This article will focus on the issue of cancer as it relates to HRT use. I will deal first with endometrial cancer, including the use of HRT in women with a past history of the disease. The rest of the chapter will deal with breast cancer and HRT, including a critical look at some of the epidemiology and an attempt to put this in perspective alongside some less well publicized observations. There are few definitive answers in this field, but it is possible to look beyond the mass of data and examine some of the underlying challenges facing researchers, clinicians and women themselves.

HRT AND ENDOMETRIAL CANCER

The detection of a marked increase in the incidence of endometrial cancer in the United States in the 1970s[1,2], following the onset of widespread use of unopposed oestrogens by menopausal women, led to a large number of reports from case-control and cohort studies. The vast majority of these demonstrated a strong statistical association between the use of such therapy and an increased risk of endometrial carcinoma. This literature has been well reviewed in recent years[3] and I will not repeat this, but there are three observations which repay closer attention. The first of these is that the relationship between the increase in endometrial cancer risk and the duration of exposure to oestrogen is cumulative, and may even be exponential. Thus, little increase in risk is detectable with therapy lasting for up to 2 years, but a very considerable increase is observed with successive years of therapy. Relative risks (RR) with long-term therapy in the range 8–15 or greater are common in the literature[4-7].

The second observation is that the increased risk associated with unopposed oestrogen use appears to persist after the cessation of therapy[5,8], in some studies remaining elevated even after 15 years of follow up[7]. This finding has implications for the long-term follow up of any woman who has received unopposed oestrogen therapy in the past, whether or not she has subsequently been treated with combined therapy. Third, although the sequential addition of a progestogen to postmenopausal oestrogen therapy can reduce the risk of endometrial cancer, probably to that of the untreated

Table 1 Relative risk of endometrial cancer with oestrogen and progesto-gen use. Adapted from Voigt *et al.*[10]

Therapy	Number of cases	Number of controls	Relative risk	Confidence interval 95%
No hormone	78	132	1.0	—
Oestrogen only	54	25	3.1	1.6–5.8
Any progestogen	18	24	1.3	0.6–2.8
<10 days/month	11	9	2.0	0.7–5.3
≥10 days/month	7	15	0.9	0.3–2.4

postmenopausal population[9,10], this protection is incomplete if the progestogen is given for fewer than 10 days in every cycle[10] (Table 1).

Taken together, these observations should strike a note of caution when we assess some of the newer forms of therapy, such as long-cycle HRT. In this form of therapy, a progestogen is administered every 3rd or 4th month, in an attempt to minimize unwanted vaginal bleeding and progestogenic side-effects. Studies of these prepara-tions lasting for 1 or 2 years have shown no increase in the inci-dence of endometrial hyperplasia compared to monthly sequential combined regimens. However, the use of this endpoint as a surro-gate for long-term safety is based on the epidemiological data al-luded to above. As mentioned, these data[10] show that even *monthly* administration of a progestogen for fewer than 10 days is associated with a doubling in the risk of endometrial cancer, raising a question mark over the long-term safety of giving a progestogen only every 3rd or 4th month. Indeed, a very recent report from Scandinavia[11] demonstrates a considerable increase in the risk of endometrial hyperplasia and carcinoma in women using long-cycle HRT. If these findings are confirmed it would be inadvisable to prescribe this form of therapy for durations longer than a few months.

HRT in women with previous endometrial cancer

Standard surgical therapy for endometrial cancer includes bilateral oophorectomy, with the result that pre- and perimenopausal women undergo a sudden loss of ovarian oestrogen secretion. Most of these women will experience severe and persistent climacteric symptoms, which do not generally respond well to non-oestrogen therapies. Because endometrial cancer is known to be highly oestrogen-sensitive, HRT has traditionally been absolutely contra-indicated in such women. Nevertheless, many women with early well-differentiated node-negative tumours have an excellent long-term prognosis. Not only are these women subjected to very disabling symptoms, they are also exposed to markedly elevated risks of coronary artery disease and osteoporotic fracture. These can be prevented by administration of HRT.

There have been no prospective randomized studies of HRT in women with a past history of endometrial cancer. Some observational series have been published[12,13]; there is no evidence for an increased risk of recurrence, some even suggest a decrease[12]. The question of whether to use a progestogen is also unresolved: theoretically, this might prevent oestrogen stimulation of microscopic areas of residual or metastatic disease. If oestrogen therapy is contemplated, it should be preceded by careful counselling of the woman (with a written statement to that effect in her notes), and should preferably be given in a specialist setting after consultation with the oncologist and others involved in her care.

HRT AND BREAST CANCER

As already stated, breast cancer is the most common concern raised by women in connection with long-term use of HRT. Based on our knowledge of 'reproductive' risk factors for breast cancer, such as early menarche and late menopause, a causal relationship is plausible. The finding of an elevated risk among nulliparous women and those with a late first full-term pregnancy, although also invoked to support the oestrogen hypothesis, is in fact related to the absence or delay of the protective terminal differentiation of breast tissue that occurs in pregnancy. Parenthetically, it is not widely appreciated that the impact of these risk factors is at least as great as any attributable to the use of HRT.

Very many epidemiological studies of HRT use and breast cancer risk have been published. The vast majority of these report either no increase in risk, or a relative risk associated with long-term therapy of less than 1.5. Most epidemiologists would agree that although case-control and cohort studies are good instruments for investigating the *possibility* that a causal association exists, they are quite poor at quantifying any such association. This is especially true of RRs with true values in the range 1.0 to 1.5, where the variation due to chance is very large in relation to the effect of therapy. This is one of the reasons why we still seem no nearer to a definitive answer than we were 10 or 15 years ago.

A detailed review of the whole literature is beyond the scope of this article and is available elsewhere[3]. I would like to present a small selection of the published studies, with the aim of highlighting some of the difficulties encountered in conducting and interpreting such work, before putting the overall findings in perspective. The studies reviewed below include one case-control study[14] and two cohort studies, one European[15] and one North American[16], along with a recently published update[17] which has received much media attention.

A US case-control study

In their large case-control study, Brinton and colleagues[14] matched 1960 women with breast cancer with over 2200 population-based controls. 'Ever' use of HRT was associated with no overall change in the risk of breast cancer. Although the RR did not reach statistical significance in any 5-year band of duration, there was a significant trend towards an increase in risk with long-term therapy (Table 2). This is consistent with our understanding of the pathogenesis of cancer. However, the increase in risk with up to 9 years' use was only 9%, and even after 20 years' use or more was much lower than the RRs of endometrial cancer associated with prolonged unopposed oestrogen use. The vast majority of women in this study had used conjugated equine oestrogens.

Detailed analysis was performed examining the effect of a previous breast biopsy (used as a surrogate for benign breast disease).

Table 2 Relative risk of breast cancer with oestrogen use – results from a large US case-control study[14]

Duration of use (years)	Number of cases	Number of controls	Relative risk	Confidence interval 95%
<5	486	640	0.89	0.8–1.0
5–9	249	259	1.09	0.9–1.3
10–14	159	141	1.28	0.9–1.6
15–19	70	74	1.24	0.9–1.8
≥20	49	43	1.47	0.9–2.3

This analysis demonstrated no increase in risk among women who started HRT before their first biopsy but a significant three-fold increase in risk among women who had taken HRT for at least 10 years after their first biopsy. Although it is an understandable omission given the number of women involved in this study, the absence of histological confirmation of benign breast disease hinders the interpretation of these data. Women with a negative biopsy may have been included in the benign breast disease category, and no distinction is made between hyperplastic and atypical forms of benign breast disease on the one hand, which are known to confer an increase in risk of breast cancer, and fibrocystic disease without hyperplasia on the other, which does not.

A European cohort study

Scandinavia in general, and Sweden in particular, has for many years given rise to important epidemiological research. This is no doubt partly due to the rigorous national systems for recording many aspects of health care, including drug prescriptions, cancer cases and deaths from all causes, thus making epidemiological studies much more viable. The Uppsala study[15] of HRT use and breast cancer is a good example. In this cohort or long-term observational study, over 23 000 women were followed for a mean of nearly 6 years. As in Brinton's study, the overall RR of breast cancer with any

138

Table 3 Relative risk of breast cancer with oestrogen use – results from the Uppsala study[15]

Duration of use (months)	Observed cases	Expected cases	Relative risk	Confidence interval 95%
≤6	23	34.5	0.7	0.4–1.0
7–36	72	65.3	1.1	0.9–1.4
37–72	53	52.2	1.0	0.8–1.4
73–108	31	24.6	1.3	0.9–1.9
≥109	29	17.1	1.7	1.1–2.7

use of HRT was close to unity. Also in keeping with the earlier study, there was a significant trend towards an increased RR of breast cancer with long-term therapy. In the case of therapy lasting more than 9 years, the increase in RR was statistically significant (Table 3).

One important reservation exists about the Uppsala study. In an analysis based on the type of oestrogen used, a significant positive trend of RR with increasing duration of therapy was seen with oestradiol compounds, but not with conjugated oestrogens or other oestrogens (predominantly oestriol compounds). Whilst such a difference seems biologically possible, it is also possible that the use of compounds containing ethinyl oestradiol (included in the oestradiol category) may be responsible for much of the increase in RR seen in this study. As mentioned earlier, ethinyl oestradiol, which was still used by postmenopausal women during the recruitment period of this study (1977–1980), is far more potent than the oestrogens currently used in the treatment of peri- and postmenopausal women.

The Uppsala study was one of the first to address the issue of combined oestrogen/progestogen therapy. The RR of 4.4 attributed to combined therapy has been widely publicized in the popular media; however, there were only ten cases of breast cancer in this group of women and the confidence intervals of the RR were extremely wide and included unity.

Table 4 Relative risk of breast cancer with current oestrogen therapy – results from the Nurses' Health Study (1990)[16]

Duration of use (months)	Number of cases	Woman-years	Age-adjusted relative risk	Confidence interval 95%
None	354	186 366	1.00	—
1–11	16	7943	1.28	0.8–2.1
12–23	16	7962	1.32	0.8–2.2
24–35	23	9787	1.44	0.9–2.2
36–59	28	13 577	1.26	0.9–1.9
60–119	62	21 625	1.62	1.2–2.1
120–179	22	9230	1.28	0.8–2.0
≥180	11	4692	1.19	0.6–2.2

The Nurses' Health Study

By far the largest study of HRT and breast cancer risk is the Nurses' Health Study. This was established in 1976, when 121 700 female US nurses were enrolled. They have been followed up every 2 years since. Unlike the studies mentioned above, the report published in 1990[16] showed no significant trend of risk, either with duration of oestrogen use (Table 4) or with increasing dose of oestrogen. These negative findings appeared to weaken the case for a significant causal relationship between postmenopausal oestrogen use and breast cancer.

How can the widely varying results from different studies be interpreted? There have been six attempts at meta-analysis of the literature, five of them published since the 1990 Nurses' Health Study report. Each applied different criteria for the inclusion or exclusion of individual studies. All but one of these meta-analyses concluded that there was no significant increase in risk due to 'ever' use of HRT. Five of them looked at long-term use, variously defined as greater than 7, 11 or 14 years' use – all concluded that this resulted in an increased risk, the summary RRs ranging from 1.2 to 1.3.

An update of the Nurses' Health Study was published recently[17]. The authors attempted to allow for the possible confounding effects

Table 5 Relative risk of breast cancer with current hormone replacement therapy – results from the Nurses' Health Study (1995)[17]

Duration of use (months)	Number of cases	Woman-years	Adjusted relative risk	Confidence interval 95%
None	972	374 197	1.00	—
1–23	82	31 966	1.14	0.91–1.45
24–59	140	49 672	1.20	0.99–1.44
60–119	150	44 112	1.46	1.22–1.74
≥120	141	37 454	1.46	1.20–1.76

of several important factors, including age, age at menopause, type of menopause, parity, family history of breast cancer and benign breast disease. Current use of HRT was associated with a significant increase in risk. In contrast with the 1990 report, there was a significant trend of increasing risk with duration of use. Moreover, the RR reached 1.46 after 5 to 10 years' use, with both confidence intervals greater than unity (Table 5). This is the first large study to show a statistically significant effect of such magnitude after this period of use. The effect of current use was greatest in older women. The increased risk attributed to HRT disappeared rapidly (within 2 years) after therapy was stopped, suggesting that any carcinogenic effect occurs late in the aetiological process. There was no evidence for a different effect of oestrogen/progestogen therapy compared to oestrogen-only therapy.

Alcohol consumption, breast cancer and heart disease

Colditz and colleagues' report[17] has received a great deal of media attention. In part this is justified, since the Nurses' Health Study is a very large and generally well-respected epidemiological project. One finding has, however, gone largely unmentioned in this country. In a separate report from the Nurses' Health Study, also published in the *New England Journal of Medicine*, Fuchs and co-workers[18] examined the effect of alcohol consumption on mortality in women. Compared to non-drinkers, there was a significant trend towards an

Table 6 Alcohol consumption among women and relative risk of death from breast cancer – results from the Nurses' Health Study (1995)[18]

Average daily alcohol intake (g/day*)	Number of cases	Adjusted relative risk	Confidence interval 95%
0	107	1.0	—
0.1–1.4	30	0.67	0.45–1.01
1.5–4.9	61	0.85	0.61–1.16
5.0–14.9	69	0.96	0.71–1.32
15.0–29.9	48	1.37	0.96–1.96
≥30.0	35	1.67	1.10–2.53

*8 g alcohol = 1 unit

increased risk of breast cancer with increasing alcohol consumption. Drinking between 15 g and 30 g of alcohol per day (approximately 13 to 26 units per week) was associated with a 37% increase in breast cancer risk, progressing to a statistically significant 67% increase with consumption of more than 26 units per week (Table 6). This level of risk is at least as great as any attributable to HRT. Alcohol consumption is not listed as one of the variables taken into account in Colditz and colleagues' analysis of HRT use and breast cancer risk, raising the question of a confounding effect. At the time of writing, this question is unresolved.

Proponents of the health benefits of moderate alcohol consumption will point to the fairly consistent finding of a reduction in death due to cardiovascular disease, particularly coronary heart disease. Indeed, this finding was confirmed in the study of Fuchs and colleagues[18], in which light drinkers (1 to 4 units of alcohol per week) were half as likely to die of coronary heart disease as non-drinkers. Even heavy drinkers (more than 26 units per week) gained substantial protection (Table 7). Of course, the same can be said of HRT: the last Nurses' Health Study report on HRT and cardiovascular disease[19] showed a 50% reduction in coronary heart disease among users of HRT compared to non-users. Thus, both alcohol consumption and HRT use may reduce the risk of coronary heart disease, and both may increase the risk of breast cancer. Somehow, in the media

Table 7 Alcohol consumption among women and relative risk of death from coronary heart disease – results from the Nurses' Health Study (1995)[18]

Average daily alcohol intake (g/day*)	Number of cases	Adjusted relative risk	Confidence interval 95%
0	145	1.0	—
0.1–1.4	47	0.82	0.59–1.15
1.5–4.9	41	0.51	0.36–0.73
5.0–14.9	50	0.64	0.46–0.89
15.0–29.9	28	0.65	0.43–0.99
≥30.0	9	0.59	0.35–0.99

* 8 g alcohol = 1 unit

reporting of these findings, the mud sticks to HRT whilst alcohol comes up smelling of roses.

The latest Nurses' Health Study report on HRT and breast cancer has prompted a reappraisal of the advice given to women taking HRT in the medium to long-term[20]. Whereas previously most experts considered that up to 10 years' use was essentially risk-free, the balance of risk and benefit in any individual woman of therapy lasting longer than 5 years is now more important. Relatively few women take HRT for this length of time; those that do tend either to dismiss the possible risks as trivial or to consider them very carefully before deciding whether to continue therapy. Women who believe that any use of HRT can increase their risk, or who have no good reason to believe that HRT will benefit them, either never take HRT or stop it after a very short duration. The views of women in the latter group are very unlikely to be changed by attempting a detailed explanation of the risks and benefits of long-term HRT use.

HRT in women with previous breast cancer

In general, the remarks made above in relation to previous endometrial cancer also apply to women with previous breast cancer. The latter is usually an absolute contra-indication to HRT, but some women with severe climacteric symptoms or strong prophylactic

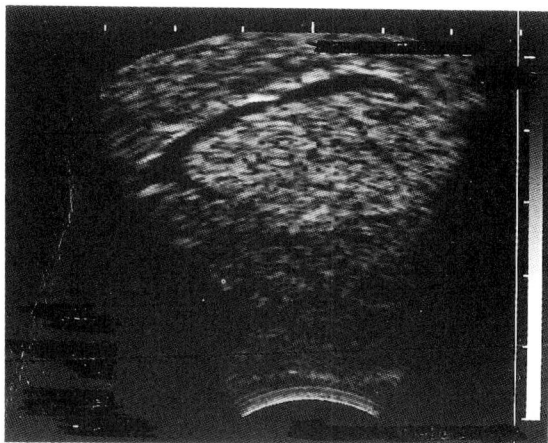

Figure 1 A large endometrial polyp identified by vaginal hydrosonography in a postmenopausal woman taking tamoxifen

indications for HRT will decide to take it, after careful counselling in a specialist setting. Observational series of breast cancer patients subsequently given HRT do not demonstrate any obvious increase in the risk of recurrence[21,22]. Again, there is as yet no evidence from randomized trials on which to base a rational approach to therapy. Such trials are planned, and a feasibility study is currently under way at the Royal Marsden Hospital in London. An essential feature of studies of HRT in women with breast cancer will be a meaningful assessment of the impact of therapy on quality of life, without which any alteration in recurrence rates or mortality will be impossible to interpret.

TAMOXIFEN AND ENDOMETRIAL DISEASE

Tamoxifen is an almost universal adjuvant therapy for breast cancer, particularly among postmenopausal women. It is considered to cause relatively few side-effects and to be safe. However, several studies have shown elevated RRs of endometrial cancer in women taking tamoxifen, including two large randomized placebo-controlled trials[23,24]. The relative risks reported were far higher than those in studies of HRT and breast cancer. Despite this, many women take tamoxifen almost indefinitely. Furthermore, trials of tamoxifen for breast cancer prevention are underway, where the putative benefits of tamoxifen therapy are much less and the risks much greater than in women with breast cancer. We should be aware of the risks of endometrial disease in such women and the difficulties involved in detecting it[25], including the common occurrence of hyperplasia or cancer in the absence of vaginal bleeding, the atypical ultrasonographic appearance of the endometrium and the frequent finding of large fibrous endometrial polyps (Figure 1).

CONCLUSION

Epidemiology will not be able to answer all our questions concerning the risk of breast cancer in women taking HRT. A large randomized placebo-controlled study might answer some of them, but this would take a very long time and the feasibility of such a study is questionable. The majority of women taking HRT only for relief of climacteric symptoms will not require therapy for longer than 5 years, within which time there should be no significant alteration in their risk of breast cancer. Women who are considering taking HRT for longer than 5 years, predominantly to reduce the risk of osteoporotic fracture or coronary heart disease, should have the most thorough assessment of their risks of these conditions available, so that the benefits of continuing therapy can be weighed against the possible increased risk of breast cancer. Finally, many women whose anxieties have been fed by scare stories in the press are greatly reassured when the figures are put into perspective alongside the many other influences on breast cancer risk to which they have been and continue to be exposed.

REFERENCES

1. Weiss, N.S., Szekely, D.R. and Austin, D.F. (1976). Increasing incidence of endometrial cancer in the United States. *N. Engl. J. Med.*, **294**, 1259–62
2. Greenwald, P., Caputo, T.A. and Wolfgang, P.E. (1977). Endometrial cancer after menopausal use of estrogens. *Obstet. Gynecol.*, **50**, 239–43

3. Mack, T.M. (1993). Hormone replacement therapy and cancer. *Bailliere's Clin. Endocrinol. Metab.*, **7**, 113–49

4. Ziel, H.K. and Finkle, W.D. (1975). Increased risk of endometrial carcinoma among users of conjugated estrogens. *N. Engl. J. Med.*, **293**, 1167–70

5. Mack, T.M., Pike, M.C., Henderson, B.E., Pfeffer, R.I., Gerkins, V.R., Arthur, M. and Brown, S.E. (1976). Estrogens and endometrial cancer in a retirement community. *N. Engl. J. Med.*, **294**, 1262–7

6. Weiss, N.S., Szekely, D.R., English, D.R. and Schweid, A.I. (1979). Endometrial cancer in relation to patterns of menopausal estrogen use. *J. Am. Med. Assoc.*, **242**, 261–4

7. Paganini-Hill, A., Ross, R.K. and Henderson, B.E. (1989). Endometrial cancer and patterns of use of oestrogen replacement therapy: a cohort study. *Br. J. Cancer*, **59**, 445–7

8. Rubin, G.L., Peterson, H.B., Lee, N.C., Maes, E.F., Wingo, P.A. and Becker, S. (1990). Estrogen replacement therapy and the risk of endometrial cancer: remaining controversies. *Am. J. Obstet. Gynecol.*, **162**, 148–54

9. Perrson, I., Adami, H.O., Bergqvist, L., Lindgren, A., Petterson, B., Hoover, R. and Schairer, C. (1989). Risk of endometrial cancer after treatment with oestrogens alone or in conjunction with progestogens: results of a prospective study. *Br. Med. J.*, **298**, 147–51

10. Voigt, L.F., Weiss, N.S., Chiu, J., Daling, J.R., McKnight, B. and van Belle, G. (1991). Progestagen supplementation of exogenous oestrogens and risk of endometrial cancer. *Lancet*, **338**, 274–7

11. Cerin, Å., Heldaas, K. and Moeller, B. (1996). Adverse effects of long-cycle estrogen and progestogen replacement therapy (Letter). *N. Engl. J. Med.*, **334**, 668–9

12. Creasman, W.T., Henderson, D., Hinshaw, W. and Clarke-Pearson, D.L. (1986). Estrogen replacement therapy in the patient treated for endometrial cancer. *Obstet. Gynecol.*, **67**, 326–30

13. Lee, R.B., Burke, T.W. and Park, R.C. (1990). Estrogen replacement therapy following treatment for stage I endometrial cancer. *Gynecol. Oncol.*, **36**, 189–91

14. Brinton, L.A., Hoover, R. and Fraumeni, J.F. (1986). Menopausal oestrogens and breast cancer risk: an expanded case-control study. *Br. J. Cancer*, **54**, 825–32

15. Bergkvist, L., Adami, H.O., Persson, I., Hoover, R. and Schairer, C. (1989). The risk of breast cancer after estrogen and estrogen–progestin replacement. *N. Engl. J. Med.*, **321**, 293–7

16. Colditz, G.A., Stampfer, M.J., Willett, W.C., Hennekens, C.H., Rosner, B. and Speizer, F.E. (1990). Prospective study of estrogen replacement

therapy and risk of breast cancer in postmenopausal women. *J. Am. Med. Assoc.*, **264**, 2648–53

17. Colditz, G.A., Hankinson, S.E., Hunter, D.J., Willett, W.C., Manson, J.E., Stampfer, M.J., Hennekens, C., Rosner, B. and Speizer, F.E. (1995). The use of estrogens and progestogens and the risk of breast cancer in postmenopausal women. *N. Engl. J. Med.*, **332**, 1589–93

18. Fuchs, C.S., Stampfer, M.J., Colditz, G.A., Giovannucci, E.L., Manson, J.E., Kawachi, I., Hunter, D.J., Hankinson, S.E., Hennekens, C.H., Rosner, B., Speizer, F.E. and Willett, W.C. (1995). Alcohol consumption and mortality among women. *N. Engl. J. Med.*, **332**, 1245–50

19. Stampfer, M.J., Colditz, G.A., Willett, W.C., Manson, J.E., Rosner, B. and Speizer, F.E. (1991). Postmenopausal estrogen therapy and cardio-vascular disease: ten-year follow-up from the Nurses' Health Study. *N. Engl. J. Med.*, **325**, 756–62

20. McPherson, K. (1995). Breast cancer and hormonal supplements in postmenopausal women (Editorial). *Br. Med. J.*, **311**, 699–710

21. Wile, A.G., Opfell, D.A., Margileth, D.A. and Hoda, A.C. (1991). Hormone replacement therapy does not affect breast cancer outcome. *Proc. Am. Soc. Clin. Oncol.*, **10**, 58

22. DiSaia, P.J., Odicino, F., Grosen, E.A., Cowan, B., Pecorelli, S. and Wile, A.G. (1993). Hormone replacement therapy in breast cancer (Letter). *Lancet*, **342**, 1232

23. Fornander, T., Rutqvist, L.E., Cedermark, B., Glas, U., Mattsson, A., Sifverswärd, C., Skoog, L, Somell, A., Theve, T., Wilking, N., Asker-gren, J. and Hjalmar, M.-L. (1989). Adjuvant tamoxifen in early breast cancer: occurrence of new primary cancers. *Lancet*, **1**, 117–20

24. Fisher, B., Costantino, J.P., Redmond, C.K., Fisher, E.R., Wickerham, D.L. and Cronin, W.M. (1994). Endometrial cancer in tamoxifen-treated breast cancer patients: findings from the National Surgical Adjuvant Breast and Bowel Project (NSABP) B-14. *J. Natl. Cancer Inst.*, **86**, 527–37

25. Ross, D. and Whitehead, M. (1995). Hormonal manipulation and gynaecological cancer: the tamoxifen dilemma. *Curr. Opin. Obstet. Gynecol.*, **7**, 63–8

10

Hormone replacement therapy: quality of life issues

M.P. Vessey, E. Daly and A. Gray

INTRODUCTION

Interest in assessing quality of life as an important outcome of therapeutic interventions has increased enormously in recent years. For
example, a *Lancet* editorial[1] on quality of life published in 1991
reported that an *Index Medicus* search for relevant papers identified
207 in 1980 and 846 in 1990. A series of articles published by Fitzpatrick and colleagues[2–4] in the *British Medical Journal* in 1992 provides an excellent summary of the use of quality of life measures in
health care.

In this article we consider the effects of incorporating quality of
life measurements into a recently-reported cost-effectiveness analysis
of hormone replacement therapy (HRT)[5].

RISK–BENEFIT MODEL

In our risk–benefit computer model, two main treatment strategies
were considered: (1) treating hysterectomized women with oestrogen-only therapy (ORT) and (2) treating non-hysterectomized
women with combined oestrogen and progestogen therapy (CRT).
Women were assumed to start treatment at age 50 with full compliance. Disease endpoints considered in the analysis included

endometrial cancer; breast cancer; osteoporotic fractures of the hip, wrist and vertebrae; ischaemic heart disease; and cerebrovascular disease. Disease risk assumptions, based on a review of the literature, were as follows:

(1)   Endometrial cancer. It was assumed that CRT users are at no increased risk.

(2)   Breast cancer. It was assumed that less than 10 years' use of either ORT or CRT is not associated with any increase in risk. Risk was assumed to increase by 30% following 10 years' use (of either ORT or CRT) and by 50% following 15 years' use, the risk remaining elevated after discontinuation of treatment for a period equal to the period of treatment.

(3)   Osteoporotic fractures. We assumed a 20% reduction in risk during the first 5 years' use of ORT or CRT followed by a 60% reduction where treatment is continued. After discontinuation of treatment, this reduction in risk was assumed to persist for a period equal to the period of treatment.

(4)   Ischaemic heart disease. Ischaemic heart disease risk was assumed to decrease by 25% following 5 years' use of ORT and 50% following 10 years' use, with risk remaining reduced after discontinuation of treatment for a period equal to the period of treatment. For CRT, we assumed a halving of the cardioprotective effect.

(5)   Cerebrovascular disease. Assumptions were as for ischaemic heart disease, but of half the magnitude.

Using the assumptions about disease risk outlined above, the computer model predicted the average life years gained per woman for different periods of treatment with ORT or CRT to be as shown in Figure 1.

QUALITY-ADJUSTED LIFE YEARS

Life years gained is not an adequate measure of outcome if health care makes an important impact on morbidity or extends life

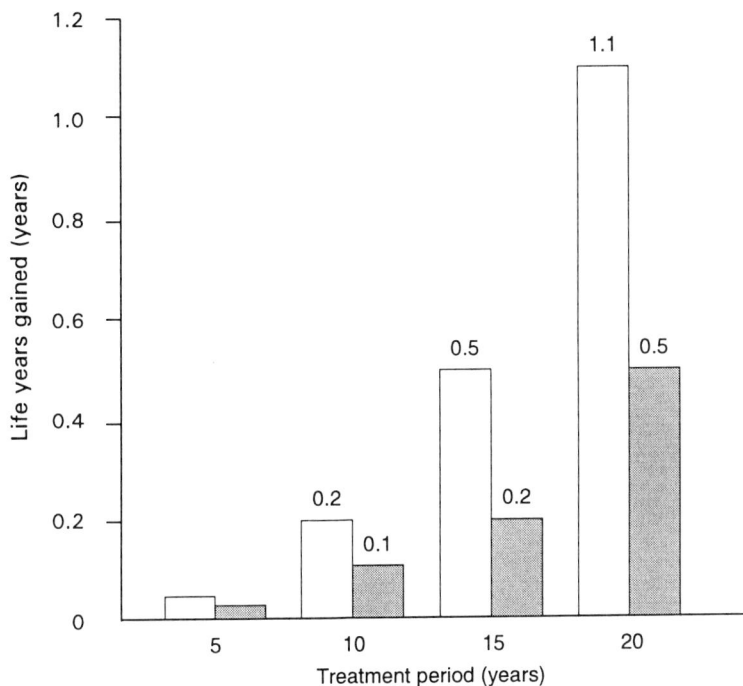

Figure 1 Average life years gained per woman for different periods of treatment with oestrogen only (open bars) or oestrogen and progestogen (tinted bars) replacement therapy

expectancy at less than full health. The quality-adjusted life year (QALY) is an attempt to address this problem. This approach involves attaching weights (or 'utilities'), between zero and one, to years of life in different health states. Thus if a treatment delays death by 1 year, but leaves the patient in pain or bedridden, then that additional life-year is weighted, so that in units of QALYs it becomes less than 1 year. Similarly, if a treatment improves physical status or reduces the duration of pain or disability, the change in weights will result in an increased number of QALYs.

The case for and against the use of QALYs in the allocation of resources has been hotly debated[6–8]. Some argue that judgements about the value of survival vs. quality of life cannot reliably be made by doctors on behalf of their patients, nor that they can be extrapolated from one patient to another. Others argue that evidence on quality of life, as well as on survival, is very important in planning health care in the current climate of cost-cutting and budgeting. The conclusion of those appreciating both the advantages and shortcomings of the QALY system is that it can serve only as an aid to, and not a replacement for, responsible discussion about the value of a treatment.

QUALITY ADJUSTMENTS FOR MENOPAUSAL SYMPTOM RELIEF

Since many women on HRT achieve relief from distressing menopausal symptoms, accounting for this improvement in quality of life is important in a full assessment of the benefits and risks of treatment. This involves obtaining utilities for health states with menopausal symptoms. A method which has been widely used in the USA for the valuation of health states is the direct 'time trade-off' method which is based on an approach developed by Torrance[9]. Using this method, the subject is offered two alternatives – a number of years (x) of life lived at reduced health (which is defined) or fewer years (y) of life lived in normal health. Time y is then varied until the subject cannot discriminate between the two alternatives, at which point the utility value associated with the state of reduced health is given by y/x. For example, a woman may consider that 10 years lived while suffering menopausal symptoms is equivalent to 8 years lived in normal health yielding a utility value of 0.8. Therefore, relief of such symptoms for a period of say 4 years could in effect be equated with an extension of life of 0.8 years (0.2×4). This extra benefit resulting from treatment must be added to the direct life years gained component to yield a quality-adjusted life years (QALY) gained figure.

In addition to making allowance for relief from menopausal symptoms, each of the diseases associated positively or negatively with the use of HRT should be taken into account in a QALY based analysis. This matter is considered in the following section.

Table 1 Assumptions used to estimate quality of life gains in relation to health effects of HRT

Health state	Utility value	Duration (years)
Breast cancer	0.80	7.5
Fractured hip	0.75	to death
Fractured vertebra	0.95	for the first 10.0 years
	0.99	thereafter
Ischaemic heart disease	0.90	5.0
Cerebrovascular disease	0.70	15.0
Menopausal symptoms	0.95	3.0–6.0*

* It is assumed that 56% of women have menopausal symptoms for 3 years, 26% have symptoms for 6 years and 18% have no symptoms

USE OF NOTIONAL QUALITY-OF-LIFE UTILITY VALUES

As a first step, utility values and their duration of operation associated with the various health effects of HRT were estimated on a consensus basis by a small group of informed doctors and other scientists. The results obtained are shown in Table 1. Quality of life gains consequent upon these estimates are shown in Table 2. The quality of life gain (discounted to present values) in relation to relief of menopausal symptoms is approximately 15–50 times greater than the gains or losses associated with each of the other health effects of HRT. Two factors contribute to this result: (1) menopausal symptoms are common and effectively relieved by HRT and (2) relief of menopausal symptoms is an immediate effect of HRT use while other effects occur mainly in the long term: discounting has the effect of reducing the present value of future events.

This exercise indicates that relief of menopausal symptoms plays a central role in the evaluation of quality of life associated with HRT use. Accordingly, we decided to undertake fieldwork to assess utility values for menopausal symptoms in a formal way rather than by relying on informed clinical judgement.

Table 2 Estimated quality of life gains per user in relation to health effects of 10 years' use of ORT (by hysterectomized women) and CRT (by non-hysterectomized women), based on assumptions shown in Table 1. Figures shown are discounted

	Quality of life gains (years)	
Health state	ORT	CRT
Breast cancer	(0.003)	(0.003)
Fractured hip	0.010	0.010
Fractured vertebra	0.007	0.007
Ischaemic heart disease	0.005	0.002
Cerebrovascular disease	0.008	0.004
Menopausal symptoms	0.147	0.147

ORT, oestrogen-only replacement therapy; CRT, combined oestrogen and progestogen replacement therapy. Figures in parentheses represent life years lost

USE OF EMPIRICAL RESEARCH TO ESTIMATE UTILITY VALUES FOR MENOPAUSAL-SYMPTOM RELIEF

Fieldwork was undertaken which involved administering a questionnaire to a sample of 63 women[10]. This sample was comprised of patients attending a specialist menopause clinic and two general practices in Oxford. The only criterion for eligibility was that women had to be aged between 45 and 60. Eligible women were given a short non-technical description of mild and severe menopausal symptoms (prepared by David Barlow on the basis of clinical experience and existing literature) (Table 3). They were then asked to indicate their quantitative judgement of the effect these symptoms would have on their overall quality of life. Two measurement methods were used: a rating scale and a time trade-off procedure. Only the latter is considered here.

Using results from the time trade-off questions, we calculated utility values relating to health states with mild and severe menopausal symptoms. For mild symptoms the figure obtained was 0.85 (95% confidence interval, range 0.80–0.90) and for severe symptoms it was 0.64 (95% confidence interval, range 0.57–0.71). We were surprised by the results obtained; clearly the women considered the

Table 3 Descriptions of menopausal symptoms

Mild menopausal symptoms may take one of the following forms:

You will have occasional hot flushes, once or twice a day, and night sweats which will wake you up occasionally. These may last for between 6 months and 5 or even 10 years.

OR

Your concentration and confidence will be poorer than a few years ago, you will cope less well with your job or other work and you will feel tired some of the time. This may last for between 6 months and 5 or even 10 years.

OR

You have noticed that your vagina is rather dry and that this makes sex a little painful. This could continue for a long time, perhaps the rest of your life. You are less interested in sex than you used to be.

Severe menopausal symptoms may take one or all of the following forms:

You will have severe menopausal flushing once or twice every hour with night sweats every night causing you to lose sleep and often causing you to change your nightdress.

You will feel very severe tiredness accompanied by a lack of concentration and confidence so great that you are failing to cope not only with your work, but also with your home life, with effects on relationships in your family.

You will experience complete lack of interest in sex which is only partly because of vaginal dryness. Your lack of interest is so great that you feel even if the vagina was not dry, you would not positively choose to have sex. This problem may be seriously affecting your marriage.

reduction in quality of life associated with menopausal symptoms to be substantially greater than members of our scientific panel had done (see Table 1). The utility values were then used to estimate average quality of life gains per HRT user. These figures allowed for the fact that a proportion of women experience side-effects while on HRT and that some women obtain no relief from symptoms. HRT has proved to be successful in the treatment of a range of menopausal symptoms in around 90% of users[11]. We therefore assumed that 90% of users experience relief from symptoms, 5% experience side-effects and the other 5% experience no change in overall quality of life. For the 5% who experience side-effects, we assumed that they remain on treatment for 6 months. With regard to duration of symptoms, it has been reported that 56% of women experience menopausal symptoms for between 1 and 5 years, and that 25% of women have symptoms for more than 5 years[12]. In the present analysis, it was assumed that on average, women experience symptoms for 4 years and that HRT users who obtain relief do so for the same period.

Adding quality of life gains associated with symptom relief to direct life years gained figures associated with the other health effects of HRT yielded average QALY gains which are shown in Tables 4 and 5. The important effect of taking menopausal symptoms into account is clearly apparent. Similarly, using financial data also collected as part of the overall project, it was possible to estimate costs per QALY; the results are shown in Tables 6 and 7. In Table 8, data are provided on estimated costs per QALY for a range of different health interventions. On this basis, the use of HRT by women with menopausal symptoms appears to provide good value for money. However, it must be borne in mind that costs per QALY for different health care interventions, derived using different methods, may not be directly comparable. Nonetheless, such comparisons may help to place the cost-effectiveness values of HRT in context with those for other health care interventions – a useful adjunct to decision making in the current climate of concern over value-for-money and uncertainty about the balance of benefits and risks of this treatment.

CONCLUSION

Quality of life may be severely affected in women with menopausal symptoms and HRT has been shown to provide relief from such symptoms in the majority of users. Consequently, it is important to include quality of life measurements when assessing the balance of benefits and risks of HRT. Existing techniques for measuring quality of life have limitations; the development of appropriate and well-validated instruments is a research priority.

Table 4 Quality-adjusted life year gains (undiscounted) associated with different periods of use of oestrogen replacement therapy (ORT) starting at age 50 by hysterectomized women with and without menopausal symptoms

Severity of symptoms	Duration of use of HRT (years)			
	5	10	15	20
Severe	1.34	1.52	1.82	2.36
Mild	0.56	0.73	1.04	1.58
None	0.04	0.21	0.52	1.06

Table 5 Quality-adjusted life year gains (undiscounted) associated with different periods of use of combined replacement therapy (CRT) starting at age 50 by non-hysterectomized women with and without menopausal symptoms

Severity of symptoms	Duration of use of HRT (years)			
	5	10	15	20
Severe	1.33	1.40	1.53	1.82
Mild	0.54	0.62	0.75	1.03
None	0.02	0.10	0.23	0.51

Table 6 Costs per quality-adjusted life year (£, 1992/93) associated with different periods of use of oestrogen replacement therapy (ORT) starting at age 50 by hysterectomized women with and without menopausal symptoms

Severity of symptoms	Duration of use of HRT (years)			
	5	10	15	20
Severe	160	270	330	380
Mild	400	630	730	790
None	14 690	5650	3740	2750

Table 7 Costs per quality-adjusted life year (£, 1992/93) associated with different periods of use of combined replacement therapy (CRT) starting at age 50 by non-hysterectomized women with and without menopausal symptoms

Severity of symptoms	Duration of use of HRT (years)			
	5	10	15	20
Severe	270	450	570	660
Mild	670	1090	1340	1490
None	40 940	19 150	13 360	9130

Table 8 Cost per quality-adjusted life year (QALY) for different health interventions (£, 1992/93)

10 years' ORT* (severe menopausal symptoms)	270
Advice by GP to stop smoking	300
10 years' ORT (mild menopausal symptoms)	630
10 years' CRT* (mild menopausal symptoms)	1090
CABG* for severe angina (left main disease)	1750
Action by GPs to control hypertension	2850
15 years' ORT (no menopausal symptoms)	3740
Breast-cancer screening programme	5550
Heart transplantation	8350

*ORT, oestrogen replacement therapy; CRT, combined oestrogen-progestogen replacement therapy; *CABG, coronary artery bypass grafting. Updated from Daly and co-workers[5]

REFERENCES

1. Anonymous (1991). Quality of Life. *Lancet*, **338**, 350–1
2. Fitzpatrick, R., Fletcher, A., Gore, S., Jones, D., Spiegelhalter, D. and Cox, D. (1992). Quality of life measures in health care. I: Applications and issues in assessment. *Br. Med. J.*, **305**, 1074–7
3. Fletcher, A., Gore, S., Jones, D., Fitzpatrick, R., Spiegelhalter, D. and Cox, D. (1992). Quality of life measures in health care. II: Design, analysis, and interpretation. *Br. Med. J.*, **305**, 1145–8

4. Spiegelhalter, D.J., Gore, S.M., Fitzpatrick, R., Fletcher, A.E., Jones, D.R. and Cox, D.R. (1992). Quality of life measures in health care. III: Resource allocation. *Br. Med. J.*, **305**, 1205–9

5. Daly, E., Vessey, M.P., Barlow, D., Gray, A., McPherson, K. and Roche, M. (1994). Hormone replacement therapy in a risk–benefit perspective. In Berg, G. and Hammar, M. (eds.) *The Modern Management of the Menopause*, pp. 473–97. (Carnforth, UK: Parthenon Publishing)

6. Cubbon, J. (1991). The principle of QALY maximisation as the basis for allocating health care resources. *J. Med. Ethics*, **17**, 181–4

7. Harris, J. (1991). Unprincipled QALYs: a response to Cubbon. *J. Med. Ethics*, **17**, 185–8

8. Wade, D.T. (1991). The 'Q' in QALYs. *Br. Med. J.*, **303**, 1136–7

9. Torrance, G.W. (1986). Measurement of health state utilities for economic appraisal: a review. *J. Health Econ.*, **5**, 1–30

10. Daly, E., Gray, A., Barlow, D., McPherson, K., Roche, M. and Vessey, M. (1993). Measuring the impact of menopausal symptoms on quality of life. *Br. Med. J.*, **307**, 836–40

11. Hunt, K. (1988). Perceived value of treatment among a group of long term users of hormone replacement therapy. *J. R. Coll. Gen. Practit.*, **38**, 398–401

12. McKinlay, S.M. and Jefferys, M. (1974). The menopausal syndrome. *Br. J. Prev. Soc. Med.*, **28**, 108–15

Index